Copyright

This book is not intended as a substitute for the medical advice of physicians. The reader should regularly consult a physician in matters relating to his/her health and particularly with respect to any symptoms that may require diagnosis or medical attention. The exercise methods and dietary methods used in this book are capable of causing significant drops in blood sugar levels. Talk to your physician before trying any of the exercise methods or dietary methods used in this book. If you are taking any medication to control blood sugar do not make dietary changes or exercise changes without the assistance of a physician, as medication adjustment will be necessary to prevent excessive lowering of the blood sugar level (hypoglycemia). Hypoglycemia from using too much medication can be dangerous.

Michael Ward is the author of one novel, four books of short stories, and thirty-five individual short stories. A complete list of his books is at the end of this book.

Michael Ward's books are published by Amazon and Barnes and Noble. Click on the link to Amazon's Michael Ward Page below to read the first part of any his books.

Amazon's Michael Ward Page   http://www.amazon.com/-/e/B007A550QM

Website: www.sites.google.com/site/michaelwardwriter

Follow me on Twitter at:

https://twitter.com/Michael56984009

I always follow back although it may take a week to ten days.

Dedication

This book is dedicated to my wife Cecilia, my children Nathan and Sarah, my son-in-law David, and my granddaughter, Avianna. No man could have wished for a better family, and I love them with all my heart.

Eastern Saying

When the pupil is ready, the teacher will appear.

Contents

Introduction

The highest blood sugar level I have had in a medical test is 293 mg/dl (16.28 mmol/L). People don't come back from that level, but I did. It took me four weeks to research type 2 diabetes, and a further eight weeks to bring my blood sugar levels back into the normal range. That was more than five years ago, and for the most part they have stayed there ever since. You probably noticed I used the words "for the most part", and that was deliberate because type 2 diabetes is like an invader in your house. You can push him out and you can build fences to keep him out, but if you drop your guard he can sneak back in. This book is about one thing, and one thing only, and that is how to balance blood sugar levels. When the Russian army used to attack in the days of Czarist Russia they would often attack from five different directions at once. An attack like that is devastating, and can easily overwhelm an enemy. Type 2 diabetes is your enemy, make no mistake about it. If you want to win, then you must attack like the Russian army from a multitude of different directions.

I was born in Scotland, which means I am descended in the most part from Vikings and Celts. The Vikings were so strong that often their enemies couldn't even lift the double headed Viking battle ax they used. One of the most famous Vikings was the Lord of the Orkney Isles. His name was Thorfinn Skullsplitter, and he typified the Vikings of his day. To a certain extent you have to think like a Viking to beat type 2 diabetes, but once you have overwhelmed your enemy, you can settle down and live a relatively normal life with only the occasional need to ride into battle again.

Type 2 diabetes is not a disease of the pancreas. I am one hundred per cent certain that type 2 diabetes starts in the liver. When you first realize that you have type 2 diabetes, your blood insulin levels are often three times normal levels. If blood insulin levels are three times what they should be, then there's nothing wrong with your pancreas. One of the big problems with Western medicine is that it looks at each organ in the body individually. Chinese medicine looks at the body as an integrated system, which it obviously is. Your body is essentially a bunch of single celled organisms, which originally banded together for mutual protection, and hundreds of millions of years of evolution later turned into creatures like us. I'm not an expert on Chinese medicine by any means, but I have books by people who are. One of the things I will look at in this book is the way in which lab rats are given type 2 diabetes for the purposes of study of the disease. The way scientists do that is to give the rats large doses of fructose, with the intention of giving them a fatty liver. Once the fatty liver is in place, type 2 diabetes follows. Does that sound familiar? In Britain, more people now get liver damage from food than they do from alcohol.

I believe I can help somewhere between 10%, and 50%, of you to throw off the scourge of type 2 diabetes. I will give you an example of the way I control blood sugar, bear with me because this example will illustrate exactly how your body stores sugar. Imagine a farmer in a dry area such as Mexico, or the Middle East 4,000 years ago. Enough rain falls in a year to grow all his crops, but the rain is variable so to make sure he always has enough water he has constructed multiple small reservoirs on his land. Water flows onto his property in four small streams, which all flow at different rates. In any one day, the streams might supply him with enough water for his crops or they might not, but over a one year period there is enough water. Given that situation, a sensible farmer will work to make sure all his reservoirs are full at all times. That way he will never run out of water, and that makes sense, for the penalties of running out of water are severe because his crops might die. So if the farmer is well organized he lives in a state where his reservoirs are as full as possible, and if the levels drop, then he fills them back up again as soon as he can. That is exactly what your body does and there is a good reason for that, which I will outline in the next paragraph.

I have read a lot of books on paleontology, and what you find in there is fascinating, and also very thought provoking. For most of the last ten thousand years the climate on this planet has been unbelievably calm, and unbelievably favorable, and that is the only reason we have cities and agriculture. For most of mankind's existence, getting enough food has been a hard task, and going for days without food has been a cold, hard fact for many of our ancestors. If your body didn't have a way to store sugar, then you would die very quickly. Sugar obviously isn't stored directly as sucrose, glucose, or fructose, but it is stored as compounds that can easily converted back to sugar. Your body stores sugar in the liver, in your muscles, and in fat, in various different compounds.

I haven't told you how I got rid of diabetes yet. I spent $300 on books, but once I realized that my insulin levels were three times higher than they should have been, I knew exactly where the attack had to be directed. My aim was to drop my insulin levels back to normal, but the only way I could do that would be to reduce the amount of sugar in my bloodstream. If your bloodstream is full of sugar then there are two things you can do. The first is to reduce the amount of sugar coming into the system, and the second is to increase the amount going out. If you change your diet to reduce the amount of sugar coming in, that will help on the input side because it means less sugar going into your bloodstream, and a corresponding reduction in insulin levels. If you empty as many of your body's sugar reservoirs as possible, that will help on the output side because your body will pull sugar out of your bloodstream to fill up its storage reservoirs. So effectively you will be going in like the Russian army, and attacking from five sides at once. Your attack will be devastating, and your body will watch helplessly as its sugar reserves begin to fall (it has no idea that there are six pizzas in the freezer just waiting to be thawed out). Your sugar reserves won't fall back to normal in 24 hours or 48 hours, what will happen will be more like a military siege and it will take several weeks. In my opinion, the body has multiple tipping points, and if you put enough pressure on the body one way or the other, then you flip it either into, or out of, type 2 diabetes. Once you flip your body out of a diabetes state, then it will stay that way, unless you change pressure on the tipping points and flip it back into a diabetes state.

This is not rocket science. It is literally an easy thing to do, all it takes is about eight weeks of persistence. Let's go back to our example of the farmer and his reservoirs. He needs a certain amount of water per day for his crops, and he has to have that. At the moment he is safe, and comfortable, with plenty of stored water. If I want to put pressure on his water storage system, all I have to do is put dams on his streams, and dig holes in the sides of his reservoirs. My dams don't have to be full dams, partial dams will reduce his water intake. The holes I dig in his reservoirs don't have to drain them completely, I can drain the reservoirs halfway down if I want. If I do that, then in a fairly short time the farmer won't have enough water stored for his crops.

Your body works the same way. If you make changes to your food intake so that there is less usable sugar or carbohydrates, then you will put pressure on input side. A simple way to do that might be to switch from simple carbs to complex carbs, which take longer to break down in your body. Switching your exercise habits to doing more exercise will start to drain your sugar reservoirs. Changing from watching television for an hour after dinner, to walking for an hour after dinner, puts pressure on your sugar storage reservoirs. Maybe they can cope if you only do it for two days, but what if you do it for two months, that's a big change to the equation.

What follows is essentially a User's Manual for tipping your body out of type 2 diabetes. It explains how I slid into type 2 diabetes, and then I go through how I pushed my body out of a diabetes state. I kept detailed records of my blood sugar levels over a four month period, and I can fairly clearly identify the point at which my body flipped into a different state. So come with me on a journey, and see if you can do what I did. The chapters in this book can pretty much be read in any order, if you wish, although reading them in the order in which they are written is probably best. Everything in this book involves ordinary food that you can buy in the supermarket, and exercises that you would do naturally as part of your daily life, if you weren't confined to a desk, or a factory, for a good part of your working day. We live very unnatural lives in this modern world, and this book is an attempt to redress some of the balance. What I did is not hard, it is actually quite easy, and really requires up to eight weeks of persistence. The methods in this book will lower most readers' blood sugar levels. They lowered mine quite drastically, and I went from a blood sugar level of 293 mg/dl (16.28 mmol/L) sometime in late October 2007, to a blood sugar level of 79 mg/dl (4.39 mmol/L) on January 18, 2008 at 5:45 pm. The level of 79 mg/dl was not an anomaly. I took eight blood sugar readings that week, and the average reading for the week was 94 mg/dl (5.22 mmol/L). No drugs were involved in those numbers, it was all exercise, diet, and pressure on tipping points that gave me this result.

Author's Note on the Spelling and Punctuation in the book

I lived in Scotland, and England, until I was 37 years old when I moved to the United States. Since I live in the United States, the English used in this book is American spelling and punctuation, in effect Webster's English. However, some spelling and punctuation may well be the Queen's English, so I apologize (apologise in the UK) in advance to anyone who is a real stickler for absolutely correct English from whatever country they are from. In places Microsoft English may also creep in as well, since I used their spell checker.

A Little History and a Journey into Type 2 Diabetes

I guess before we start, I better tell you a little about myself. I am just an ordinary man. My background is accounting and finance, and cost engineering. I have had an interesting, and somewhat different life than many people. I was a single father for six years; I brought my son up on my own from age eight months old to age seven, and my son still lives with me now. I have driven fifty miles on the frozen surface of the Beaufort Sea north of Alaska. I did that on my own in a Ford F150 truck without anyone with me and I can recommend it as a life experience. I've been in temperatures of minus 85 fahrenheit (minus 65 celsius) with wind chill, and I've walked five miles (eight kilometers) in temperatures of plus 95 fahrenheit (35 celsius) on many occasions. I've never been to war, but my grandfather lied about his age and arrived on the battlefields of World War I aged either fourteen or fifteen years old. They wouldn't let him fight but they did let him drive an ambulance on the battlefields, and he probably knew more about the horrors of war than most men. His job was to pick up wounded men and get them to the medical areas. My father was eighteen years old in 1942. He had some damaged fingers and was excused from going to war by the military doctor. He told the doctor he could fire a sub-machine gun and asked to go. The doctor gave him three chances to say no, and after the second time he said he was going the doctor told him that he had one more chance to say no. He said he was going for a third time so the doctor sent him to war. My grandfather was unaware of all this and thought my father would be excused. When he found out what my father had done, he swore for one of only three times in his life. My father didn't talk about the war much, but he did tell me once that he was down to lead a squadron of men in the invasion of Japan. If America hadn't dropped an atomic bomb on Japan, he would very likely have died somewhere in Japan, along with millions of other British and American soldiers sometime in 1945 or 1946. 451,000 British people were killed in World War II, or about 1% of the British population. To put that into perspective, the Russians lost the most people in World War II; 26.6 million Soviet citizens died or about 13.9% of their population.

That last part didn't necessarily tell you a lot about me, but what it did do was lead to me growing up in an unusual generation. I was born in Scotland, in 1959, and most of the people I went to school with had fathers who were in World War II, and there were a lot of tough kids around. I remember when I went to the grammar school, there was one kid three years older than us on the bus who used to lie on his back on the seat on the upstairs deck, pull his knees up to his chest, and then kick out as hard as he could at whichever one of us was going past him. The best way to pass was to be second in line, and shoot past as he was drawing his legs back to kick the next one. He usually got the first, and the third one, but he didn't get me too often, when he did you felt it. Years later it occurred to me that if the four of us had gotten together, we could have all attacked him at once and overwhelmed him, even though he was a lot bigger than us.

I used to play chess a lot at school. I always used to play an attacking game, and I used to win most of the matches. One kid once said that he preferred to play me rather than anyone else because I never played the same game twice. I remember my father taught me to play chess when I was six years old, and I remember sitting at the board on my own at age six practicing moving the knight around the board, and being fascinated by the way it could move. When I was a teenager I was once in a hopeless position at chess and another kid advised me to resign. Even though I felt instinctively that this was wrong I did so, but I spent the rest of the day feeling like I wanted to throw up. I realized there was something inherently wrong about resigning at chess and I have never ever resigned since. I have no problem with another person resigning, and I have no problem being beaten at chess, but I am mentally incapable of resigning. I feel so strongly about this that I told my son never to surrender if he is ever in a war, and I also told him that if his commanding officer ever orders a surrender, then he should shoot that same officer in the back of the head. The average European army will turn and run when 55% of the men are dead, but apparently Scottish armies have often fought on when 85% of the men were dead, and maybe my views have something to do with that.

One of the things that happens in Britain or it did when I was young, is that a certain proportion of kids get quite bad acne, the type that will lead to facial scarring. When I was twelve years old I went to a cousin's wedding, and saw a teenager who was about eighteen years old who was in quite a bad way. At the time there were four classes with 30 kids in, making 120 of us and I had the worst case of spots out of the group of 120 (this should not gross you out because there is a point to it, and that point concerns willpower, and the ability to connect seemingly unrelated facts). I realized that if I had the worst case at age twelve and that was consistent month by month, then by the time I was eighteen I would almost certainly have facial scarring. I resolved to find out what caused teenage spots and acne and was surprised to find out that nobody actually knew, including my parents. Sugar seemed to me likely to be the obvious cause, but every article in the newspapers said it wasn't. While I was reading up on this I was also observing, and I noticed there was a three day time lag between eating sugar and spots appearing. I decided then and there to give up eating sugar, and also to give up eating anything with sugar in. Sugar isn't routinely added to everything on the supermarket shelves in England like it is in America, so this was actually fairly easy. I allowed myself sugar on Christmas Day and maybe on my birthday, but I told my mother I no longer wanted fruit pies, custard or anything with sugar in. I kept this up for more than five years between the ages of twelve and seventeen, and only started eating sugar again sometime in my eighteenth year. It worked because slowly over time I went from having the worst case of spots out of the 120 of us to moving up the rankings, and by the time people were at the age where you can get facial scarring I was relatively free from spots, especially the ones that could cause scarring. To an American this may seem odd, but there was a huge amount of pollution in Britain at the time from all the factories, and I suspect the combination of dust particles and moist air made things worse.

I guess what I'm trying to say here is that if a twelve year old can give up sugar for five years, then you shouldn't have any trouble doing it for a couple of months. The kind of willpower I use does not come from aggression, but is more a kind of quiet determination. A man who is sufficiently determined can often achieve far more than a man who is aggressive because the aggressive man will only annoy people, whereas the quietly determined man will often just keep going until he succeeds. There is an American called Marc Allen who is about ten years older than I am. I have never spoken to Marc Allen, but I have quite a few of his books and he has the same kind of quiet determination that I do. He is the owner of the New World Library, and at age thirty he was unemployed, broke, and struggling to pay the rent on his small apartment. He resolved to start and run his own business despite having no start-up capital, and six years later at age thirty-six he was a millionaire. Most of this was due to quiet determination, and it would be of great benefit to our society if more people used quiet determination to succeed, rather than aggression and trampling on others.

When I grew up there wasn't a lot of money for fast food and coke. Water was served with school lunches. I took sandwiches, and occasionally you would see one kid with a can of coke, but that didn't even happen every day. My parents were middle class, and most of the kids in the grammar school were middle class. Many of our parents had been children during the great depression, and they had a natural instinct not to waste money. Just so you can see the kind of food I grew up with, my school lunch always consisted of three slices of white bread with one slice of ham, or cheese, in between the bread plus an apple. That was all I ate between breakfast, and dinner time. I think there is a lot to be said for that, the French don't snack between meals, and their heart attack rates and general health are much better than the heart attack rates in Anglo-Saxon countries. In fact, a French man is actually less likely to have a heart attack than a British woman is, even though both countries have very similar cholesterol rates. French heart attack rates are quite close to Japanese heart attack rates, which are way lower than West European and North American heart attack rates. Statistics like that are worth mentioning, and instead of referring to it as "the French paradox", American researchers should be swarming all over France trying to find out why their heart attack rates are so much lower than ours. They are obviously doing something right that we are not, or alternatively, we are doing something very wrong that they are not. Last time I checked, America and Britain tied for sixth place for heart attacks, despite the fact that all the Statin drugs Americans take are supposed to prevent heart attacks.

I mentioned what I ate at school just to give someone a contrast between what is eaten now, and what was eaten then. A schoolchild now can look forward to a totally different menu than a schoolchild had before 1980. I remember going through the school cooking area once, and it was full of school staff peeling vegetables like carrots (when did your child last eat a real carrot), potatoes, peas, and other vegetables. The women who worked there had real jobs, and real wages, unlike the minimum wages staff like that earn now. That is more than thirty years ago now, and when schoolchildren ate food like that they just didn't get type 2 diabetes. There are other factors, of course, like lack of exercise, and I will go though those during the course of this book. This idea of shipping in food at minimal cost didn't exist when I was growing up, it came into existence in the 1980s. I remember saying at the time that cost cutting would destroy the West because one of the first things to go in a cost cutting environment is R & D, and unfortunately I have been proved right. In 1980, the West was light years ahead of the rest of the world, not so now. There is actually more gene sequencing capacity in just one building in China than in the whole of America, and one of the reasons is that university budgets have been stripped to the bone. If we were still operating on the methods we used in the 1960s, and 1970s, then every university in the United States that wanted a gene sequencing machine would have one. The next super weapon to be invented may well be an RNA virus, and we would do well to change the way we fund our universities back to the way we funded them before the cost cutting era began. Of course, this book may well end up all over the world since type 2 diabetes is now a global epidemic, so if you are reading this book in Asia you well have a different take on what I just said. One thing that concerns me is that our politicians in the West are now making many of the same mistakes that were made in ancient Greece and Rome. Don't any of them know the value of reading history books?

I went for a five mile walk after writing the last section. It was cold, but I did it anyway because that is what I do with exercise. I have found that if you just have a vague plan to exercise, it doesn't work. The only way it works for me is to say that I am going to exercise five days a week, and then just do it. If you drop one day, before you know it you're dropping two, and then a few weeks later you realize that you are only exercising one day a week. I don't usually exercise at weekends, although I do use them as a catch up time if need be. If it rains I will usually just go anyway, unless it is a major thunderstorm. I used to live in England, and if you're not prepared to go out in the rain in England, then you will never exercise. You may wish to walk in the mall, but I prefer fresh air. Today it was 56 degrees (13 celsius), which for me living in Florida is nice, more often than not it is close to 90 degrees (32 celsius), and that tends to be too hot. I plan to cover exercise in more detail in a separate chapter, but I just wanted to let you know what I did today. Later I may do some forward and reverse wrist curls with a barbell, and I may do exercises to work my biceps and triceps. You can do 100 forward wrist curls on each wrist fairly quickly, which tightens your whole wrist area and also gives you a strong grip. I will describe the weightlifting exercises I do in the exercise section. I like free weights because you are much less likely to injure yourself, and you have a lot of control over which muscles you want to work.

You may say to me that you don't have the time to walk five miles, and my answer would be to ask if you have time to watch television for an hour and a half a day. If you do, then you have time to walk five miles. There is a direct correlation between the amount of time a person watches television and their chances of getting type 2 diabetes. Given the state of American television these days, it's not as hard to give up as it would have been fifty years ago.

It occurred to me earlier that I had made an analogy to an attack by the Russian army, and some Americans may be wondering why I hadn't made an analogy using an attack by US forces. The reason I didn't do that is that an attack by the US tends to involve a lot of noise and sudden heavy explosions, followed by total devastation, and that is not the sort of war we are fighting here. This is more of a war of attrition where your enemy is tough, and you starve him out. You can't just drop a large bomb in this case, you have to attack from all sides, use ambushes wherever necessary, and if you catch your intruder anywhere near the top of the stairs then you push him backwards down the stairs, run after him, and jump on his head. This is what it's going to be like, sometimes you'll catch him at the top of the stairs, other times you will see him approaching from an upstairs window, and have time to run down and intercept him. Another time you might catch him with his fingers on the fence at the edge of your property, about to climb up, and all you have to do is smash his fingers with a hammer. Each time you push this guy back through, you can put up more defenses, and each time you catch him sneaking in you learn, and in theory he shouldn't be able to sneak back in the same way.

You don't have a sub machine gun that you can use one time to blow your enemy away. Your defense is to continually drain your body's sugar reserves faster than they can fill up, and once you get good at that you can live a fairly normal life. Far too many people today rely only on their pancreas to correct a high blood sugar level, and that is the reason so many people are getting type 2 diabetes. Far too many people are working their pancreases far too hard. If you are stuffing your face with cookies all night, then your pancreas is working far harder than your grandfather's did. You need to rest the pancreas if you are not going to trash it. In the old days, many people walked after dinner, and if you do that then you pull sugar right out of your bloodstream to give you energy for the walk. Do that, and suddenly your body goes from working to clear sugar out of your blood, to checking whether it has enough sugar in your bloodstream for the walk to come. Your body will also learn from exercise, if it knows that you are going to go for a walk every day after dinner, then it will be prepared. Remember also that what I did when I started trying to reduce my blood sugar was to aim to reduce the amount of insulin in my blood, that comes first, and reducing blood sugar levels is a side effect of that. In the early days I always aimed to be exercising within fifteen minutes of finishing my meal. Of course, there are only certain exercises you can do that soon after a meal. You can walk, but you can't lift weights. If you can walk up an incline so much the better, but don't go for a steep hill. Use your common sense here.

One thing I am not going to do in this book is dwell on the negative things that can happen with type 2 diabetes. In my opinion fear is not a good motivator, and just leads to additional stress. There seems to be a need by advertisers in the United States to sell products based on the use of encouraging fearful thoughts, and that really is not good for people or for society in general. One of Churchill's great statements during World War II was that there was nothing to fear, except fear itself. Fear is not a motivator at all, it tends to paralyze people rather than motivate them. If there is something I do which I think may be useful, then I will tell you because I am a great believer in the American saying that nobody should have to reinvent the wheel.

Sliding into Diabetes

I don't necessarily like the title I used in this section, but it does give an accurate impression of what happens. While I was out walking yesterday I was thinking about this section, and how to write it, and one of the things that came into my head was that type 2 diabetes does not search you out, you search it out. Let me explain what I mean by that statement. Type 2 diabetes is currently hovering over the human race like a cancer. More people are getting type 2 diabetes now than at any time in recent history. It is not just Americans, it is all over the world now, and it seems like no area is safe. I read last year that diabetes rates are skyrocketing all over the Middle East, both in Muslim countries and in Israel.

In the next section I am going to talk about tipping points that can flip you into type 2 diabetes. Type 1 diabetes is likely caused by a virus. I remember reading years ago in England, that there are peaks in type 1 diabetes at age four when children first go to school, and again at age eleven, which is when children go to secondary school and are exposed again to new groups of children. In type 1 diabetes, the part of the pancreas that pushes out insulin is destroyed, whereas in type 2 diabetes the pancreas still puts out insulin. Type 2 diabetes develops over time, type 1 diabetes develops suddenly.

I found out that I had a blood sugar rate of 293 mg/dl (16.28 mmol/L) sometime in October 2007, and I can identify at least three tipping points that were going on during that summer. At the time we were putting in a new computer system at work, and I was working a lot of extra hours on that. I remember working quite a lot of weekends, and also working late into the evening. I can remember sitting on the back deck of our house on a summer evening with a book, and thinking I should go for a walk to get some exercise, but I was just too tired. I was probably too tired to cook much that summer too, which means that I was eating in restaurants far too much.

To go back to what was going on with me that summer, I was also not getting enough sleep, which encourages insulin resistance, and not getting enough sleep is another tipping point. One thing I will say to governments right here and right now, is that if you create conditions where you neglect the health of your citizens, then over time you risk invasion by another country because you will fall behind other countries. It is very unlikely that the United States will ever have to fear invasion by another country, but it is quite possible for Europe, given the massive changes that are going on around the world right now. A transfer of wealth from one area of the world to another is almost always a recipe for chaos, and having a population where everybody over fifty is on six different tablets makes you less able to withstand the pressures of the modern world.

In the summer and early fall of 2007, I was also flying to different areas of the southeast region of the company I was working for, and I remember having several nosebleeds while I was out at plants in the Mississippi area. This had more to do with the dry air and the dust at the plants I was going to, but I didn't know that so I checked in with my doctor. I found out that my blood pressure was above normal, and that was probably caused by excessive insulin in my blood. When I arrived home from the doctor's, I was talking with my family. I was frustrated that I could have high blood pressure at the age of only forty-eight. Now if you are an American, and you think that everyone over aged forty should expect to have high blood pressure, then think again because there are many areas of the world where people in their forties don't have high blood pressure. There are way too many Americans in their twenties and thirties on blood pressure medication, and if we don't get a handle on that then the next generation will just regard it as normal.

My step-daughter came into the room as I was telling my wife and son about the blood pressure reading at the doctor. I was telling her about it, and I made some comment that it would be just my luck to have high blood sugar as well, and I ended up asking her to check my blood sugar. I expected it to be normal, and my intention was just to make sure it was normal, but it came out at 255 mg/dl (14.17 mmol/L). I didn't know exactly what the numbers for normal blood sugar readings were, but I did know enough to know that anything over 200 mg/dl (11.11 mmol/L) was probably not good. I asked if she could check my son's blood reading too, which was a classic case of clutching at straws. He was seventeen at the time, and his reading was 87 mg/dl (4.83 mmol/L), which is pretty much where a reading should be for someone his age. I went out for an immediate walk because I figured I could walk it off. I know all the distances of all the walks around my area now because I measured them in my car, so I walked 1.9 miles. When I got home I asked Sarah to check my blood sugar again, fully expecting a significant drop. It had dropped, but only ten points, and it was now 245 mg/dl (13.61 mmol/L), which was still way too high.

The doctor had asked me to get blood work done by the end of the week so I exercised each night, confident I could pull it down. I had the blood test taken later in the week, and was told they would call me if there was anything wrong, but otherwise I would get the results when I went to see the doctor the next week. One to two days after I had the blood work done, I arrived home from work to find a message on my answering machine telling me to call the doctor straight away about the results of my blood work. I called, and the test had indicated that my blood sugar was 293 mg/dl (16.28 mmol/L) on the morning it was taken. This was not the best news, I had gone in just a week or two from not having any health problems to appearing to have some major problems.

I have always been a believer in the fact that your problems do not go away if you ignore them, so I went out to Barnes and Noble and looked at their books on diabetes. I bought two books and began reading, but I didn't feel like I was getting enough information. Although the Scots make up only 5% of the population of the UK, they are responsible for 15% of the inventions made in the UK, and many of those inventions are great leaps forward. I have always said that if you put any of my cousins on my mother's side in a lab, and gave them enough funding, they would invent something useful. My father's family is very intelligent too, but my mother's family has inventive brains. I was very good at jigsaw puzzles using more than a thousand pieces when I was young, and I still do a lot of thinking using the same principles that you use to put a jigsaw puzzle together, whether at work or when facing a problem outside work. Often I would have pieces on the board that didn't necessarily connect, but looked as though they fitted in a certain area, and if you do that your subconscious mind learns to see patterns that aren't immediately obvious to the conscious mind. I read the books I had bought at Barnes and Noble, but I felt that all I had done was scratched the surface, and I was struck by the feeling that there was a lot missing from the board. I was in exactly the same position as I was when I was confronted by the fact at age twelve, that if I didn't do something about the spots that were appearing on my face, then I would have scars by aged eighteen. Some part of my mind felt that there was an answer in there somewhere, if I could only find out more information. Since Barnes and Noble just didn't have enough books, I went on Amazon. I was lucky, I had a good job, and I saved a portion of the money I earned, instead of just blindly spending everything so I was in a position to shell out $300 for books on Amazon. Not everybody can do that, and if I hadn't had the spare money at that point, then this book would not have been written.

Within a few days, boxes of books started arriving from Amazon. I have always been a fast reader, so I started working my way through them. As I read the books, my mind started putting pieces into place on the mental jigsaw puzzle I was carrying in my head on type 2 diabetes. I had already been exposed to diabetes in the house, with my step-daughter having type 1 diabetes. The first thing my wife did when my son and I moved to America was to show me a syringe in the fridge which contained a glycogen injection, and she explained what to do if Sarah's blood sugar dropped unexpectedly. We have never had to use that syringe, but there are plenty of parents of small children and teenagers who have had to use it, and there are also plenty of husbands, and wives who have had to use it on their spouses. This is just a magnified version of what your liver does all the time. Since I worked out how to drop my blood sugar, through diet and exercise, I have had occasions when I have arrived back from a heavy exercise session, taken my blood sugar, and gotten a reading of 79 mg/dl (4.39 mmol/L) or 80 mg/dl (4.44 mmol/L). A reading of 80 mg/dl is right at the bottom of the normal range, and there is no doubt that at that point my liver intervened and released glycogen into my bloodstream to push blood sugar back up. One of the reasons type 2 diabetes is giving us so much trouble at the moment, is that the human system is primarily focused on coping with low blood sugar caused by having too little food, rather than high blood sugar caused by having too much food. One thing you also need to remember is that humanity has spent most of its existence living a nomadic existence, and it is inconceivable from a point of view of evolution, that a human would spend most of the day in a sedentary position such as at a desk in an office, standing at a machine in a factory, or sitting in front of a television. The average modern man has way underdeveloped muscles compared to a man living a nomadic existence ten thousand years ago, and when I say man, I mean women too, try walking ten miles with a twenty pound toddler in your arms, and you will see a significant drop in blood sugar, and your arm muscles will get a good workout too.

I said a paragraph or two ago, that I spent $300 on books with Amazon. One of the books that came in the mailbox was a book about the first year of having type 2 diabetes. This one book was instrumental in making me absolutely determined to fight type 2 diabetes. It was a book written about the first year of having type 2 diabetes. I'm sure the author meant well, but the main message of the book was that you just had to accept you had type 2 diabetes and get on with it, and there was an overwhelming message of futility in the book. I just don't believe you should blindly accept anything that makes your life more difficult, and I have to say that if the Founding Fathers had taken that attitude, then America might well have remained under the control of London for another hundred years.

Somewhere in all the reading I came across the point that when someone first gets type 2 diabetes, their insulin levels are typically three times normal. Like I said before, it is patently obvious that if the pancreas is churning out enough insulin to hold levels at three times what they should be, then the problem is not in the pancreas. Once I put that piece into the jigsaw, it created a lot of interconnections. The first conclusion I came to was that the cause of type 2 diabetes could not possibly lie in the pancreas, it had to be somewhere else. The fact that the pancreas was working so hard meant that it needed to have the pressure taken off it, so my first aim was to get the insulin levels in my blood down. This ought to be a foregone conclusion, in the same way that you keep your heart strong by working it harder than it normally needs to be worked, so that it has extra capacity for when you inadvertently put pressure on it.

I remember that I started from the point of view that the first thing I needed to do was to get my insulin levels down, and from there I came to the conclusion that I needed to both lower the amount of sugar getting into my blood, and I also needed to step up the amount of sugar taken out of my blood. That would take the pressure off my pancreas, and it could surely cope with the rest. Remember your body is a giant reservoir that holds as much sugar in storage as possible. Empty that reservoir, and excess blood sugar will go to fill that reservoir up.

There you have it, this is the essence of what I do. I have been doing this for five years now. Due to the fact that I live in a very unnatural world, as do most of you, I have to do things that would just be done naturally. If I lived ten thousand years ago, then I would be living as a nomad, and I might walk five to ten miles a day looking for food. At the end of the day, I would have to pitch my tent, or yurt, or whatever, and that would also burn up calories. I would probably have eaten while I walked, which would mean mostly raw food. Raw food is a complex carbohydrate, and is harder for the body to burn than cooked food, which again would mean less sugar entering my system and more burned off, and note here that I use the terms sugar and carbohydrates interchangeably. If I had caught an animal during the day, then I would cook it at night, and to catch that animal I may well have to have chased it down, again burning a lot of blood sugar. Homo Sapiens Sapiens, which is us, tended to hunt small game, Homo Sapiens Neanderthalensis tended to hunt large game, and probably had more organized hunts than our ancestors did. We know that from the bones around the campsites. Bread and writing are inventions of cities, and it is unlikely a nomad would have had access to anything like bread. Ten thousand years ago, all my tools would have been made of stone, and I would have carried those with me everywhere I went. One of the main causes of type 2 diabetes may well not be spelt "s-u-g-a-r", instead it may well be spelt "c-a-r", or "c-i-t-y".

One more point, and then we will move onto the next section. My doctor is excellent as are most American doctors. I have lived in two countries, and American doctors are well trained, and if there is a major problem they will usually spend a lot of time with you trying to find that problem. I do want to say though, about two years before I discovered I had type 2 diabetes I had a different doctor, and I remember saying to him that I felt like something was out of balance in my body. I am an observant person, I can tell by the sound of the engine in my car whether it is low on oil or not, and I have been able to do that with all my cars. Perhaps this is a bad example, and everybody can do that, but if you can't do it, then there is a slight change in the tone of the engine when it is not well lubricated. If I can tell when my car engine needs oil, and it is not even part of me, then I should know when something feels different in my own body. However, when I told this to the doctor I had at the time he gave me a strange look, and I have to ask why he did that. If I had said the same thing to a Chinese doctor he would have swarmed all over it, and asked me multiple questions. If you read books on Chinese medicine, then sometimes a problem in one organ may be caused by an imbalance in another organ.

I will leave you with one thought to close this chapter. I do not know a lot about martial arts, but I can see that their development owes a lot to a way of thinking that just does not exist in the European or North American mindset. Although white people are perfectly capable of learning martial arts, and some Europeans and Americans are very good at them, nothing like that has ever existed in thousands of years of European culture, and I don't think Europeans could ever have developed martial arts. Before you blindly dismiss this comment out of hand, just think about it. Could we in Europe or North America, at our level of development, have considered the focused use of force directed into certain parts of the body? A huge number of inventions have come out of Europe and North America, but I don't think it is in our mindset to think of our bodies in the same way that Asians who speak tonal languages do. I think we can learn a lot from that.

Tipping Points for Type 2 Diabetes

Bear with me on the next few paragraphs because I am going to use tipping points on the Earth as an example to move into discussing tipping points in our bodies. If you read books on paleontology then one thing you will come across is tipping points. Every planet or moon in the solar system with an atmosphere or volcanism, or both, is subject to tipping points. Saturn's moon, Titan fascinates me because it has lakes of methane and ethane, and it also has rain falling in the form of methane and ethane. It would be a good place to look for life in this solar system just because of the constantly changing conditions. I don't think we are going to find complex life on Titan, but we might easily find some kind of single celled life.

Dig down far enough on Greenland, and you can find that it once had a tropical rainforest and crocodiles. Go back thirty million years, and you can find a black layer in the chalk deposits in Europe that was once part of the bottom of an ocean. That black layer in the chalk tells us that the ocean it came from was devoid of oxygen at the time the layer was laid down, and the black layer is made up of the bodies of millions of sea creatures that died and fell to the bottom of the ocean, but failed to decompose. Planetary tipping points abound, and oxygen levels on the Earth can vary between probably as low as 13%, and probably as high as 28%. The ancestor of the dinosaurs evolved at a time of mass extinctions, when oxygen levels on the planet may well have dropped down to as low as 13%. It was the only land creature of any size that made it through the mass extinction, and it was nine to ten feet long (three meters). The dinosaurs had the best lungs any creature has ever evolved on this planet, and their descendants, the birds can breathe unaided at heights that would kill a human.

We now have ice cores that go back up to 200,000 years from different parts of the planet, and we can cross check these with other records. What those records tell us is that the Earth can flip very fast into alternative conditions. In one part of the ice cores, the descent from warm conditions into an ice age took place in as little as ten years, with most of the temperature change happening in the first year. Whatever caused that was some kind of tipping point because there was a major change in temperature in just one year. It is looking more and more like the Earth has multiple tipping points, many of which have positive or negative feedbacks, and what is also increasingly obvious is that a minor change in one place on the planet, may cause a much more magnified change somewhere else on the planet.

I suspect that we are in the same situation with our bodies. I think our bodies can be flipped into, and flipped out of, type 2 diabetes by what are sometimes quite minor changes. My grandmother developed type 2 diabetes sometime in her seventies. In those days, if you were going to get type 2 diabetes, it usually happened at that kind of age. It did not happen at twelve years old like it does now, so we have changed something in the mix. It was perfectly possible to get type 1 diabetes at age twelve, or at age four, or age eight, but it was extremely rare to develop type 2 diabetes at that age. Type 2 diabetes used to be called "adult onset diabetes" for a good reason, and that reason was that it only happened to adults. I remember when I was at university in Nottingham, England. One day I was talking to a student who I didn't know that well, and he told me that he had developed diabetes. I knew a little about type 1 diabetes, and I assumed that was what he had, but it wasn't, he had type 2 diabetes. He was in his early twenties, and he was slim. For some reason we expect people who get type 2 diabetes to be overweight, but that is not always the case. There is a couple we know in Jacksonville, who have both had type 2 diabetes for around ten years. They are both slim, but they eat out every single night. In their case that is the trigger, although I suspect that lack of exercise also plays a part.

I read a report written about a professor who was training medical students in the United States. One day his students told him they didn't like dissecting old people, and asked if he could get them some young cadavers to work on. As a reader you may have comments about this, but this request produced some valuable information. The professor was able to procure cadavers from traffic accidents, who had volunteered their bodies for medical research. As you would expect for Americans in their twenties, the bodies were in very good shape physically with very few problems. However, there was one thing the professor noticed, and that finding was consistent with just about every cadaver they dissected. Although the bodies were from people in their twenties, the livers in just about every single body were more consistent with a cadaver aged between seventy and eighty.

Something has changed obviously. Many people in both America and the UK are now eating terrible diets, and I will cover this far more in the food section, but what I do want to say is that there may be multiple tipping points right there, just in the liver.

A couple of years ago my wife and I took a trip to the North Carolina and Tennessee Mountains to see the fall leaves. One of the places we went to was Dandridge, Tennessee. Dandridge has been there a long time, and is in a beautiful setting. Five men who fought in the Revolutionary War against the British were buried there, and one thing that was really interesting was how long they lived. I'm going to mention their names here, just in case anyone wants to look them up, and I will mention their years of birth and death, and how old they were because they lived longer than American men do today. The first one was John Blackburn, who was born in 1741, and died in 1808, which would make him 67 years old. Abednego Inman was born in 1752, and died in 1831, making him 79 years old; Samuel Lyle was born in 1747 and died in 1834, making him 87 years old; Richard Rankin was born in 1756 and died in 1827, making him 71 years old and Samuel Rankin was born in 1738 and died in 1828, making him 90 years old. The average age of these five men when they died was 78 years old, which is exactly how long an American man can expect to live now. For some reason we are told that people lived short lives until relatively recently, but that is just not the case, although if you go back to the late 1800s and the twentieth century, you will find men living shorter lives. So in 200 years of industrialization we are now back to where started with life expectancy, only I suspect modern people are much sicker and much less well nourished. These men obviously survived smallpox, diphtheria, typhoid, and all the other infectious diseases or they would have died younger, but what this shows is that a man who avoided disease could live for a long time. The difference is probably that they didn't have to work away in factories or offices, which has to decrease life expectancy even if only due to stress. By the way, people worry these days about the fact that nobody is immunized against smallpox. If you catch a disease called cowpox, you will be

28

immune to smallpox. Don't try this at home, but it is worth knowing in an emergency. Edward Jenner noticed in the late eighteenth century in England that milkmaids always had good complexions, and that was because they didn't have smallpox scars. When he investigated, he found out that all the unscarred milkmaids had gotten cowpox at some time in their lives. You get cowpox from cow udders when you milk a cow, which is why you never hear of it now. Once Jenner realized that, he began inoculating people with the cowpox virus, and within a generation he had wiped out smallpox in England.

Let's look at tipping points now, and we will start with your working life. The more hours you work, the more likely you are to develop insulin resistance, which is a major tipping point for type 2 diabetes. I suspect that if we plotted hours worked per year against incidence of type 2 diabetes, then we might see a correlation. Things are only likely to get worse if you have to go in at weekends. When I was young in Britain, it was pretty much expected that you would go abroad for two weeks and lie on a beach or go skiing. I know quite a lot of Americans who have never had two weeks off at once. What I used to find was that the first week would be spent recovering, and the second week you would really relax. I used to come back from these two week breaks incredibly relaxed, and my company benefited because I would feel like Superman for at least thirteen weeks after I got back. It is quite possible that the reason we never invent anything of any great worth in America anymore is because everyone is so tired all the time, and we have to stop that because it will really kick us in the face if we are not careful.

Lack of sleep is another major tipping point. Insulin resistance can develop very quickly if you get less than eight hours sleep a night. I remember in Britain in the 1980s, when people suddenly had to be busy all the time because that was what you had to be. At first a lot of people pretended they were busy, but now it has become a mindset, and now everyone really is busy. Thousands of years ago our ancestors had time to look at the moon, and work out that there was an 18.6 year lunar cycle called the "lunar standstill". We know that, because they built it into the layout of the stone circles that they built all over Britain. They also built Pythagoras triangles into the stone circles, and that was at least 1,000 years before Pythagoras was born. We are unable to pinpoint exactly when the stone circles were built because we can't date them, but interestingly, I saw a program on television saying that the land that is now the Yorkshire Moors was once farmed so intensively that it ruined the land, and now you can't grow crops on it. I would bet that the intensive farming was done to feed the men who built the stone circles, and if we can pinpoint when the Yorkshire Moors were farmed so intensively, then we have a potential date for when the stone circles were built.

Another tipping point is definitely how much processed food you eat. I cook most of my own food. I will give you a few recipes to start with later in the book, and most of them will take less time than it takes you to get in your car, drive to a restaurant, order, eat and then drive home. The recipes will consist of vegetables you buy in the supermarket, herbs, and Indian spices, and of an appropriate protein source such as meat or fish. Just eating a real vegetable, instead of the crap that a food corporation serves you, will have an almost immediate effect on you, especially on your energy levels. I once heard a young guy in a gym say to the trainer that he wasn't building muscle as fast as he expected. The trainer was experienced, and asked him two questions, how much sleep are you getting, and are you eating vegetables? I wasn't surprised by the first question, but I was interested to see a trainer tell the young guy that he would build better muscles by eating vegetables. Studies have shown that men who eat a salad every day for lunch in Britain are only half as likely to develop type 2 diabetes as men who don't, and I presume the same is true for women.

One of our most serious problems in America today is that although many people are overweight, they are suffering from malnutrition because there are no micronutrients in the processed food they are eating. All the vitamins are probably gone too, although they will have added vitamins made in a lab to the mix. If you eat only processed food, and I peel and grate a raw carrot, eat a raw tomato, and eat a lettuce leaf, then I may well take more micronutrients in that one quick snack than you get in a month. Our bodies work by using numerous enzymes, which go through multiple processes. A lot of those enzymes need micronutrients to run, and if the appropriate micronutrient is missing, then the conversion being done by the enzyme will just stop, and your liver will pick up the pieces and clear whatever it is out of your blood stream. In addition, you will not get the benefit of what the enzyme was trying to make. If you are tired all the time it is quite likely you are just missing micronutrients, and we have no idea what missing those micronutrients does to us. It could be the difference between needing glasses, and not needing glasses, or it could be the difference between having type 2 diabetes, and not having it.

There is something called the "twenty year rule", which says that twenty years after white flour, white bread, and white sugar are introduced into a country, rates of type 2 diabetes skyrocket. Although we are advised in America to eat a lot of whole grains, I am not sure they are much better for us. Grain products can deliver a lot of sugar into your blood stream very quickly, and you should certainly be wary of this. I remember, when I was a child, grandmothers would often say that pasta, white rice, and bread would make you fat. I remember when I was in my early twenties, my father would always have a slice of buttered white bread with his dinner. I started to do the same thing, and had to stop doing it because I started to put weight on. That was the only thing I had changed in my diet, so it was obvious that bread was causing the weight gain. An Indian man I worked with a few years ago told me that Indians often have very high triglycerides (in the 500 mg/dl range or above), and that this is caused by eating a lot of basmati rice, which is a white rice common in Asia.

A major tipping point is how much exercise you take, or much more likely, how little exercise you take. Exercise is a major tipping point, and when I told you that I attacked from five directions at once like the Russian army, then exercise played a major part in this. There is a whole chapter in this book devoted to exercise. Attacking with exercise will put massive pressure on the tipping points that can tip you out of type 2 diabetes. Once your blood sugar numbers are normal again, if you were to keep everything else the same and vary your rates of exercise, you would be able to see the effect of different amounts of exercise on your blood sugar numbers. I spend quite a bit of time exercising, and I am sure if I just decided to do no exercise for one month, and spend exactly the same amount of time sitting in front of the television, I would clearly be able to see the difference in my blood sugar numbers as they started to rise again.

Another tipping point is stress, and at the opposite end of the spectrum, your ability to relax. Reduce stress where you can. Everyone has different lives, and so everyone has different things that stress them. Some of them are similar and follow common patterns, and others are unique to a specific individual. I have covered relaxation with some unique ideas that will dovetail into whatever you already do in that area, but a key thing here is the balance between relaxation and stress. Try to push the balance more towards relaxation, and as far away from stress as you can. Obviously that is easier said than done, but if there is anything you can change then it will likely pay enormous dividends.

One very interesting tipping point is glucose transporters. Many of you may not have heard of those, since the first one was only discovered in 1988, but basically they are transporters that move glucose around the body, and there are ways that you can affect the efficiency of the glucose transporters in your body by the use of natural methods such as increased exercise. GLUT 4, or Glucose Transporter 4, is the main glucose transporter we will be concerned with when we discuss glucose transporters. This is the one that is involved with transporting glucose into muscles. I will go through a study done at the Washington University School of Medicine in St. Louis, Missouri back in 2006, which basically covered the effects of stimulation on muscle tissue, and the effects of glucose transport into muscles. There are different ways that muscles can be made more sensitive to insulin, and the path we will be looking at is exercise. Next time you go to your local fast food restaurant, take a look at the young jock who is scarfing down a meal that would push your blood sugar sky high. One of the reasons he can get away with this, and you can't, is that the glucose transporters in his muscles are likely responding better to insulin than yours are. More on that, and how to change it, in a later section.

The other tipping point I'm going to look at, is not so much something that can tip you into type 2 diabetes, but something that can help tip you out of it. Yoga and Tai Chi both claim that they affect the energy meridians in your body, and that practice of either of them can help certain illnesses. Western science cannot measure anything like energy meridians, but I would like to look at this in more detail. More on this in a later chapter too. Now we need to take a look at how I climbed out of a blood sugar level of 293 mg/dl (16.28 mmol/L), and into normal territory between 80 mg/dl (4.44 mmol/L) and 126 mg/dl (7.0 mmol/L). I did that by putting pressure on the tipping points for type 2 diabetes, and that is the subject of the next chapter.

Climbing out of Diabetes

I think the most important decision I ever made in my life was to aim to reduce the insulin levels in my blood, rather than reduce the levels of sugar in my blood. You might say, well, what's the difference? Reduce one and you reduce the other, and to a certain extent that is true. However, if you are aiming to reduce insulin levels, then that means you have to be exercising as soon as possible after you have eaten because the longer you wait, the more your blood sugar levels will rise as the food you have eaten is digested. If you just aim to reduce your blood sugar levels, then maybe you will wait longer. That also meant that I was thinking along the lines of heavy exercise, rather than just walking, although I did do both.

You have to go in hard when you first start. That doesn't mean you exercise like crazy on the first day, or you'll spend the next week unable to do anything. What it means is that you find something that is easy to do, and then do a lot of it. If you can lift a thirty pound weight, then try doing a lot of lifts with a fifteen pound weight, and work your arms to exhaustion without straining them. There is far more information in the exercise chapter so please do not try any exercises until you read that. When I say go in hard, what I really mean is that during the first eight weeks your exercise levels will be higher, and your food consumption will be tighter than you need to have them later.

I kept detailed records of the exercises I did, and detailed records of where my blood sugar levels were. Sometimes I checked my blood sugar four times a day. If you think your fingers hurt, then think of American soldiers in the conditions they have to be in now. Pricking your finger is nothing compared with they go through. If you are not American, then think of the soldiers in your own army, for every country has fought a war at some time or other. My generation didn't whine or complain because our fathers had marched across Europe, and some of them didn't make it back. My father had an uncle who lost an arm in World War I. When my parents talked about when they were young, my mother might mention a man's name, say that he had been a good dancer, and then say that he was killed in France or Germany during the war.

That didn't just happen a few times. They knew a lot of men who had died, and they also knew women who had been left widows. The father of my first girlfriend was shot down over Germany. He was put in a POW camp, but he escaped, got out of Germany, and made it back to England. As soon as he made it back to England, the first thing he did was get back into a fighter aircraft and fly back over German lines.

I just pulled up the excel spreadsheet I used to record all my blood sugar readings back in late 2007, and the first half of 2008. Your blood sugar machine can give you some records of blood sugar readings, but I spend most of my working life on excel, and I can do a lot with it, including going directly into visual basic to write macros. In one place I worked at back in Washington D.C., they were spending forty minutes a day, two or three times a week, changing the views manually on a huge spreadsheet with multiple tabs. I spent one afternoon writing them a macro, which took me maybe an hour and a half. After that all they had to do was press one button and it did that forty minute job in less than fifteen seconds, so I saved them almost an hour and a half every week. They also did the changeover much more often because it took fifteen seconds instead of forty minutes, and if they added a new project, I went right into visual basic in the macro and altered it. I didn't go on a course to learn how to go into visual basic, I just went into it, read the lines of code, and figured out how to alter it myself. It wasn't difficult. If a macro you have written fails, then you can usually figure out how to fix it by looking at where it stopped working.

I said all that to say that if you know how to use excel, then set up a spreadsheet or if you wish, email me at the email address at the end of the book, and I will send you one you can use. You will be able to study your blood sugar readings far better on excel than by pulling them up on your blood sugar meter. The value of excel, and keeping records, is that you can look back and see if you are exercising less. Maybe your average blood sugar readings for the week went up. I used to keep an average for each week of morning readings, and an average for the week in general. You can pick out trends, for example, I have said elsewhere my blood sugar reading on a Monday morning was almost always higher than on a Tuesday morning. Why was that? I already know the answer, but if

I look at my records I would see that I ate out over the weekend, and I didn't exercise on Saturday or Sunday, but I exercised Monday to Friday. On Monday I would be back to my exercise and diet routine, and I would have prepared my own food Monday night. By Tuesday morning I had dropped my blood sugar back again. Now this trend would have appeared after the initial period, when I got my blood sugars under control. For the first few weeks, my blood sugar readings were all over the place, with some good and some out of the region between 80 mg/dl (4.44 mmol/L) and 126 mg/dl (7.0 mmol/L).

I started exercising on November 22, 2007. By the morning of Monday January 7, 2008 my readings were mostly in range, so it took me maybe six to seven weeks. Perhaps I could have done it quicker, but we went to Aruba over Christmas, and that blew me out of the water because I had no control over what happened during that week. However, something like this is interesting because I can see from the numbers that they were starting to go down by the time I went to Aruba, but it was like I lost a week or two of control and slipped back a little bit. Make sure you keep a record of every blood sugar reading you take, and make a note of anything out of the ordinary because sometimes the bad readings can tell you a lot. Having said that, my first reading in the 80s was after a lot of exercise in one evening. The next night I did no exercise at all, and the reading I had was 60 mg/dl (3.33 mmol/L) higher. That reading, of course, was over the limit, and what is more the one the next morning was also over limit. Something like that immediately tells me the power of exercise. Once I realized that exercise could have such a big impact I knew that I could get things under control because a change of 60 mg/dl (3.33 mmol/L) from one night to another was massive. At that point, I think I was still draining my blood sugar reservoirs because as I got more into it, the big swings between readings just disappeared, and they were all good. Remember what I said earlier about tipping points, I think that sometime in those first eight weeks I overwhelmed type 2 diabetes, and I flipped out of a diabetes state, and you can see it in the numbers.

I am going to go through the numbers week by week. I won't go through every number, or I will bore you to death, but I want to give enough detail, so that the people who really want to see a progression can see it. Please write to me at the email address at the back of this book and give me feedback about this section because I can change it in just a few hours and republish it. The book should be electronic at first, and then available as a paperback soon after, and I can make changes to both copies and republish. I would love to hear from you. I would far rather be reading letters from readers than reading the news, and I reply to every email I receive.

I said earlier that I went to the doctor sometime in October 2007, and when the results came back my blood sugar level was 293 mg/dl (16.28 mmol/L). My step-daughter Sarah had done two readings a few days earlier, the first showing 255 mg/dl (14.17 mmol/L), and then an hour later, showing 245 mg/dl (13.61 mmol/L) so I knew I had a problem. It was hard for me to actually take my blood sugar at that point because I knew the numbers were going to be bad, and it is quite possible I just didn't want to see them. I don't want to dwell on this, but I didn't take the first reading until Saturday December 8, 2007. I have checked my exercise records and I started exercising on November 22, 2007. On that evening I walked 4.3 miles. By then I had driven in my car, and measured the distances for all the possible walks that could be done from our house. From that distance, I can even tell you exactly which walk I did that night. I am lucky in that I can leave my house and walk. Not everybody can do that, but if you don't have to drive then you save time.

I stepped up the walking pretty quickly. By the end of that week, I had walked 14.8 miles. The following week I walked 16.5 miles, and in week ended December 9, which was when I first took my blood sugar I walked another 16.0 miles. You can see by these numbers that I already had an attack in place on my blood sugar levels. In three weeks, I had walked 47.3 miles. This is 47 miles I didn't walk in the previous three weeks. That's a lot of energy burned, and to do that I pulled sugar out of my bloodstream to power all the muscles I used. When you're walking, you tend to breathe faster and deeper, which also increases energy burned. There is nothing here that you can't do, 47 miles in 21 days is an average of 2.3 miles a day. I had the flu from Monday December 3 to Wednesday December 5, which means I did no exercise those days. I played catch up later in the week, and on the Saturday I walked 8.0 miles. Once again, read the exercise section for more advice on exercise, and how to build up to this, and always check with your doctor before starting any exercise program.

Up to that point, I had mainly concentrated on walking, although I had done a little stair climbing. On Saturday December 8 I climbed 10 flights of stairs, and I did the same on the Sunday. I may have done this because Saturday was the first day I took my blood sugar on my own. It is highly likely I wanted to get some exercise in before taking it because I didn't check my blood sugar level until 3:27 pm on the afternoon of Saturday December 8. It was 120 mg/dl (6.67 mmol/L). Now this number still indicates that I had a problem with blood sugar, but it was just within the limit, and it was a heck of an improvement on a morning blood sugar level of 293 mg/dl (16.28 mmol/L) from late October. A number like this would almost certainly have given me hope that I was on the right track, but at that point I still would not have known whether I could succeed or not. I took my blood sugar again that evening at 6:59 pm, and it was 108 mg/dl (6.0 mmol/L).

Now let's see what exercise I did on that day because you can be sure those numbers were helped by exercise. That was the day I walked 8 miles, and that probably had a lot to do with me plucking up courage to take a blood sugar reading. I also climbed 10 flights of stairs. Now just to get one thing clear, I do not need to do anything like that now. That was the week I was sick. I have since read that if you are sick your body pumps extra sugar into your blood, and I think I remember having blurred vision while I was sick, and that probably stressed me a little. I have never had blurred vision since then, but that was probably me trying to exercise the sugar out of my blood. For that day at least, I succeeded in getting readings that were in the normal range, and that is a good start.

It's quite likely I went to bed on Saturday night feeling like I had made some progress. I took my blood sugar four times on Sunday, and that day turned out to be a whole different ball game, and this is what you are going to see in the first few weeks. I had good days and bad days. Let me give you the blood sugar numbers first, and these are for Sunday December 9, 2007; 11:30 am 126 mg/dl (7.0 mmol/L); 12:16 pm 136 mg/dl (7.56 mmol/L); 5:36 pm 115 mg/dl (6.39 mmol/L); 10:08 pm 134 mg/dl (7.44 mmol/L).

This is a prime example of what happens while you are working on draining your blood sugar reservoirs. The day before I had two blood sugar readings that were both within the 80 mg/dl (4.44 mmol/L) and 126 mg/dl (7.0 mmol/L) limits. On the Sunday, despite exercising a lot, two of the readings were over the limit, one was bang on the upper limit, and only one was inside the limits.

Let me tell you what I did with exercise that day, but don't get discouraged because the readings were bad because what I was doing was putting pressure on my blood sugar reservoirs, and at the same time I was strengthening my muscles as you will see from the workout, and I was also working on the glucose transporters in my muscles.

On that day I walked 5.6 miles, I climbed 10 flights of stairs, and I did the following weight lifting exercises; 80 forward wrist curls (80 on each wrist), 50 reverse wrist curls, 50 concentration curls, 40 single arm extensions, and 20 side bends. Each number means that those lifts were done on both arms or both sides. This is quite a lot of exercise, and the numbers were still bad, but this is a waiting game and a war of attrition. Remember when I told you that you have to think like the Russian army in Czarist Russia, and attack from five sides at once. Well that is exactly what I was doing here. I attacked by walking, I attacked by stair climbing, and I attacked by weight lifting. That's an attack on three sides. I was also attacking with food, but I hadn't really fully developed my strategy at that point. There will be more detail about what I did in the food section, but if I see any notes at the side here I will tell you because one of the later ones does indicate why at least one reading was higher. One note on food here though, if you have cereal or milk at night it will tend to push up your blood sugar. Milk pushes sugar into your blood over a period of hours during the night, and cereal will dump it in pretty fast. Do not ever eat cereal that has sugar added to it in the early days. Once you have control you can maybe do that later, and I can't say I have not eaten that but it is certainly not something I would eat every day. I don't buy cereal with sugar in but my wife does, and very occasionally I will have some of hers, but it might be literally once every couple of months. This day was a Sunday too, so it is quite possible that my wife and I may have gone out to eat, and I can't say for sure, but if we ate out then there would be more carbs in the food than if I cooked my own food.

What I am going to do next is have a date header for each week, so if you get tired of reading, you can just skip ahead, and there will be a conclusion at the end of this section. None of the other sections will be like this, in that we are almost plowing through statistics, but I feel this will help people who feel that this can't be done because you will see a week by week improvement, and it will also help you if you feel you are having setbacks because you will see the same things in my numbers. However, once I had been at this for a few weeks the numbers started to level out, and many more of the numbers were in the right region between 80 mg/dl (4.44 mmol/L) and 126 mg/dl (7.0 mmol/L), and after Sunday January 6, 2008, I only had two numbers out of the limits. These were a reading of 127 mg/dl (7.06 mmol/L) at 6:22 am on Tuesday January 29, 2008, and 130 mg/dl (7.22 mmol/L), on Tuesday February 12, 2008 at 6:25 am. It is interesting that both occasions were Tuesday mornings, I just took a look at the Tuesday in between to see if that was high relative to the other mornings, but it was actually 100 mg/dl (5.56 mmol/L), and that was the second lowest reading of that week, and I had all seven mornings recorded.

The morning readings are the hardest readings to bring within limits. A lot of people have trouble with this, but let's think again and apply common sense, and not necessarily look at it from the perspective of science. When I was young, my father once told me that when my sister and I were little, he would wake up every time he heard a noise in the house but as we got older this faded away. We live in a fairly safe, secure world these days, at least from the point of view of wild animals attacking us, but for most of the millions of years of our ancestry we had to be prepared to leap into action at a moment's notice first thing in the morning, or even during the night. Now how would we do this if our blood sugar was low? I suspect that our bodies are geared up to have a ready supply of blood sugar on hand for when we wake up, and if this is the case, then it is no wonder that blood sugar tends to be higher first thing in the morning. On the spreadsheet I have a separate tab with just the morning blood sugar readings on it, and I also have a week by week average. I just took a look at that, and I'm going to list it below, and you can see it drop week by week until it gets into the normal range, and then it just stays in the normal range. I only have numbers on the spreadsheet until the middle of April 2008, but I do remember things getting a little crazy at work around that time.

I am going to list the week ended and the average for the morning blood sugar readings for each week. What you will see is that by week ending January 13, 2008, the average readings were well inside the normal range at an average for the week of 107 mg/dl (5.94 mmol/L). Although I have this as a table on the spreadsheet, I can't put it as a table here because I will be converting the word file to a "web page, filtered" file for upload to Amazon and Barnes and Noble, and that will strip out the table formatting. However, I will list them line by line, and you will get the general idea:

Week ending 12-16-07; average morning reading 172 mg/dl (9.56 mmol/L)
Week ending 12-23-07; average morning reading 127 mg/dl (7.06 mmol/L)
Week ending 12-30-07; average morning reading 137 mg/dl (7.61 mmol/L)
Week ending 01-06-08; average morning reading 134 mg/dl (7.44 mmol/L)
Week ending 01-13-08; average morning reading 107 mg/dl (5.94 mmol/L)
Week ending 01-20-08; average morning reading 101 mg/dl (5.61 mmol/L)
Week ending 01-27-08; average morning reading 102 mg/dl (5.67 mmol/L)
Week ending 02-03-08; average morning reading 103 mg/dl (5.72 mmol/L)
Week ending 02-10-08; average morning reading 103 mg/dl (5.72 mmol/L)
Week ending 02-17-08; average morning reading 112 mg/dl (6.22 mmol/L)
Week ending 02-24-08; average morning reading 106 mg/dl (5.89 mmol/L)

Week ending 03-02-08; average morning reading 104 mg/dl (5.78 mmol/L)

Week ending 03-09-08; average morning reading 104 mg/dl (5.78 mmol/L)

Week ending 03-16-08; average morning reading 105 mg/dl (5.83 mmol/L)

Week ending 03-23-08; average morning reading 94 mg/dl (5.22 mmol/L)

There are no results for week ending March 30, 2008, and there is a note about going on a trip to Georgia with work, and coming back tired from the trip. The next few weeks I appear to have been taking readings sporadically, and it looks like things were probably getting a little crazy at work because I know the crash of 2008 was almost upon us at that time, and a lot of our plants were not doing so well. You can see from these average readings though, that up until week ending January 6, 2008, the readings were not really in range, but after that they were pretty much all in range. This backs up what I said about tipping points, and flipping your body into or out of type 2 diabetes. Sometime between week ending January 6, 2008, and week ending January 13, 2008, I think I flipped my body out of type 2 diabetes. It looks as though it happened suddenly.

Actually I was just looking at the numbers, and there is something really interesting here. On Sunday January 6, 2008 there is a note that I stopped drinking coffee and began drinking Japanese green tea instead. That is really interesting. I am an accountant and I am trained to pull information out of the numbers, and that is definitely significant. It is sitting there right in the numbers, and I am writing as I discover it (I have been doing this all my working life like this). I think the tipping point was close, but I think the change from coffee to green tea may have pushed things over the edge, and pushed me out of a diabetes state. Coffee tends to push your blood sugar numbers up by an average of about ten points, and green tea is said to be a very healthy drink. Now do not assume that all you have to do is drop coffee and drink green tea, I think from the numbers that the green tea just hastened a tipping point that was close to fruition, and maybe brought it forward one week because the numbers were already dropping. In week ending January 6, the reading for Thursday January 3 at 5:58

42

am was 128 mg/dl (7.11 mmol/L); Friday January 4 at 6:25 am was 142 mg/dl (7.89 mmol/L); Sunday January 5 at 9:45 am was 131 mg/dl (7.28 mmol/L) so these three readings were all over the limit.

On Monday January 7 at 6:20 am it was 120 mg/dl (6.67 mmol/L), which is within limits but still quite high. On Tuesday January 6 at 6:20 am it was 109 mg/dl (6.06 mmol/L), and on Wednesday January 9 at 6:22 am it was 97 mg/dl (5.39 mmol/L), and on Thursday January 10 at 6:25 am it was 93 mg/dl (5.17 mmol/L). Now another interesting point here was that the night before the two readings in the 90s, I had eaten mahi mahi fish with broccoli, which means very little actual carbs were consumed both nights, as broccoli is a complex carb. These two meals are an example of increasing the attack to four different directions. On the exercise front, I was attacking in three directions with weight lifting, stair climbing, and walking, and on the diet front the meal eaten at night was just fish and broccoli, which drops very little sugar into your bloodstream. I remember I pretty much settled on fish and broccoli, or fish and brussels sprouts, for the next few weeks although later I would have fish with my vegetable soup recipe, or the vegetable soup with brown rice for dinner. I think what I did here was to just wear down the level of sugar in my blood sugar reservoirs, and I suspect that I also increased my muscle strength, meaning that my muscles were pulling more sugar out of my bloodstream. By the beginning of week ending January 13, 2008, I pretty much had things under control. I still had to work hard, but by then nearly all my readings were inside the limits of 80 mg/dl (4.44 mmol/L) and 126 mg/dl (7.0 mmol/L).

As I have said in this book on several occasions, I am just an ordinary man. If I can do it then you can do it. Quiet determination is the key to this. If I face an obstacle, I put my head down and push harder, and it usually pays off. Just push, push, push, and you will win through.

I think at this point, I may well have written enough for this chapter. I will put an appendix at the back of the book (Appendix 1), with much more detail about the first few weeks. Although I said the switch to Japanese green tea was right on the tipping point at January 6, 2008, I think that just hastened things by one week. I would suggest trying Japanese green tea anyway just in case it did help. I buy mine in Costco, and it is made by a Japanese company called "Ito en". You can also buy it on Amazon, and here is the link which will allow you to see a picture:

http://www.amazon.com/dp/B000WB1YSE/

The other change here was that I also switched to eating fish and leafy greens at night, and that means there was very little carbs in my evening meal. That too would definitely have put more pressure on my blood sugar levels. As I have said earlier in this book, each chapter is a standalone chapter. Read the chapters on exercise and diet and apply them. I hope that what worked for me will work for you. I am certain I can pull a good number of you out of type 2 diabetes, and I hope to hear from you by email once you begin to apply the techniques in the book. Remember to check with your doctor before trying any of the methods to lower blood sugar, especially if you are on any medications for blood sugar. Appendix 1 covers each week in detail with analysis and explanations of what I was doing, and it would be probably be very beneficial for you to go through that section, but it is far too long to include in the main part of the book.

The Joys of Exercise

I called this chapter "The Joys of Exercise" because if you do it right, exercise is a joy. The part of my day when I exercise is often one of the most relaxed parts of the day. If I'm not relaxed when I start exercising, then I'm always relaxed by the time I finish. I exercise outdoors when I can, and that depends a lot on personal preference and on what part of the world you live in. I spent a good part of my early life in England, which meant that it often rained. If you live in England, and you are not willing to walk in the rain, then you will not have much of a life in my opinion. Some days in England I walked for six to eight hours in constant rain, and as long as I had the right weather gear then I was fine. I once hiked to the top of Mount Snowdon, which is the highest mountain in

England and Wales at a height of 3,760 feet (1,146 meters). Six weeks later I did it again, only this time I took my six year old son, and my French au-pair. I walked it first on my own to ensure that it was safe for a six year old, and it was, and then I told my son, Nathan, that if he could walk to the top he would be the only child in his class who had done something like that. There is actually a restaurant on the top of the mountain, and a train track up to the top built by the Victorians so no matter how much of a struggle it is to get there, a climber always knows that at the top he or she can sit in the warmth and buy fresh sandwiches and coffee. Nathan told me when he reached the top that he had been a little tired but had not wanted to tell me, which was something I hadn't thought of, but he still remembers that day now so it left him with good memories.

One of my close friends, David Roe introduced me to hiking, and he did it because he could see that as a single father with an eight month old son, and a job as a Controller for a German multinational that I was actually under quite a bit of stress. At first I was reluctant to go hiking, and Dave made several attempts to persuade me to go, but it was the best thing I ever did. I still remember a lot of details of that first hike, we actually hiked for 13 hours, but we were both around thirty-one years old, and both in good shape. Dave had several different versions of the hike planned in case I got tired, but it was such a wonderful day and the hike took place in such a great area, that I just didn't want to stop. It was a clear blue sky day in May, which is rare in England, and it was warm but not hot, so it was perfect hiking weather. We hiked together a lot over the next six years until I left England, and I have many great memories of those days. Dave was, and still is an interesting conversationalist, and we had many great conversations, but at the same time we also had part of the hikes where we hiked separately, each lost in his own thoughts, which was also very relaxing. Dave planned all the walks because he had the time, and I would always make all the sandwiches for the hike, and provide the soft drinks. Doing it that way allowed us to spend the whole day on a hike instead of having to stop somewhere to eat, and many times we ate sandwiches looking at an absolutely amazing view. I have so many incredible memories from my times with Dave that I couldn't even begin to list them all, and we went all over the country, taking in Scotland and Wales as well as many remote parts of England. We have stood on the ramparts of huge castles in Northumberland, which were built to protect against Vikings and Scots, and we also once hiked on the Western Isles in Scotland after an incredible five hour ferry ride across Scottish waters that were as flat as a millpond, on a beautiful Scottish day. Anyone who has ever sailed those waters will probably think we had the only calm day in a century because those are some of the roughest waters in the world. The woman we stayed with on the Isle of Barra told us about one trip when the ferry left for the mainland, and the waters were so rough that every single passenger on the ferry except her got off at the first island they came to, and refused to get back on again. I used to know a Scottish woman called Anne, and she and her husband Robin used to hire a seventy foot sailing yacht with another couple, and sail those waters in the summer, and she told me it took a lot of skill to sail in those waters. When we were on Barra we took a small tourist boat to several islands to the south of Barra, all of which are uninhabited now except for birds and sheep, and that was certainly a memorable day.

I used the example above just to show what can be done with exercise. Exercise can be taken in many different ways in many different settings, and what you have to do is find an exercise that is good for you. I am not a big fan of the "no pain, no gain" philosophy, in my opinion that just leads to injury. I have done all kinds of exercises over the years. In the exercise part of the book I will also talk about yoga and Tai Chi, as well as conventional forms of exercise. Many of you may not know this, but Tai Chi is developed from a set of exercises that were originally used in China to strengthen the body for martial arts training, and a Tai Chi session can be extremely strenuous. One thing we just do not pay attention to here in the West are energy flows around the body. Just before the collapse of the Soviet Union, a group of Russian scientists were experimenting with using a galvanometer to check electrical fields at all the body's acupuncture points. I don't remember the details fully of their research, but the Russians were able to use these measurements to predict disease, and they claimed a 70% accuracy rate. This is something that needs to be put under serious investigation. Both yoga practitioners and Tai

Chi practitioners claim that energy flows in the body can be realigned, and opened up again by doing their exercises, and this is something that should be investigated.

We have a blind spot in the West, in that we assume that, unless something was developed by Western scientists then it has no value, and that is an attitude of mind we need to get out of. Most of the drugs we use in the West were originally given to us by shamans living in the forests in remote areas of the world. At present we really do not have a proper understanding of the processes that cause type 2 diabetes. We can clearly see the end result, but the cold, hard fact is that somehow during the last thirty years, we have changed one factor, or more likely a range of factors, that has tipped us into a situation where type 2 diabetes is much more prevalent. It may be diet, it may be lack of exercise, or it may be a problem with nutrients. Farm the land long enough, even with crop rotation, and you will destroy the nutrients in the soil. Do not imagine that wheat grown on the Prairies now has anything like the nutrients in it that wheat that was planted when the Prairies were first plowed over, had in it. When we lived in Alaska, we took the cable car up to the ski area on Mount Alyeska. Sometime in the early 1950s the American ski team trained at Mount Alyeska, and there is a black and white photograph of the team. Those young Americans look so healthy that they look like Greek Gods and Goddesses. Young athletes do not look like that now, they may have bigger muscles, but they don't have that healthy, clean cut look that young Americans had in the 1950s.

Besides yoga and Tai Chi, I also want to look at a range of other exercises. Working out in a gym or at home is important. There is something called "muscle memory", and that means that once you have developed muscles in an area one time, it is then much easier to develop muscles again in the same area. When I first had high blood sugar I realized that I needed a hard exercise, a normal exercise, and exercises with weights to increase the rate at which I pulled sugar out of my body. I am a great believer in doing exercises that follow the natural movements of the body. For example, if you are out for a walk then walk normally, rather than doing exaggerated swings of the arms. Some books will tell you that this burns more calories, and perhaps it does, but it may also put strain on your shoulder joints. Humans have unusual shoulders in that our shoulders are shaped differently than most mammals, and this is due to an evolutionary niche filled by the Great Apes. If you look at a baboon on all fours what you will see is a dog with a monkey's head, whereas if you look at a chimpanzee on all fours you see something entirely different. The reason for this is that the chimpanzee's shoulders, along with our shoulders and those of the other Great Apes, are designed for climbing trees vertically by clinging to the trunk of the tree, rather than swinging from the branches. This adaptation allowed apes to get to areas that monkeys were unable to get to as easily, and it also allows an ape to weigh much more than a monkey because he or she uses the trunk of the tree to gain height, and not the branches. It would be interesting to look at the DNA listing for the design of a monkey's shoulders, and the DNA listing for the design for an ape's shoulders just to see where the differences are. I am fascinated by DNA and what it tells us. We know, for example, that Fiji was colonized by people from Papua New Guinea. We also know, from analysis of the mitochondrial DNA of the people of Fiji, that most of the original women colonists from Papua New Guinea came from the lowlands, but we know that 18% of the people of Fiji are descended from women from the highlands of Papua New Guinea. We know that when Neanderthal Men moved from the Middle East to Europe they developed red hair, and the gene for red hair on the Neanderthal chromosome is in a slightly different place than the gene for red hair on our chromosome, although it is in the same general area.

DNA analysis allows us to trace the genetic history of the people who live in on the islands in the South Pacific. The island of Fiji was once a Polynesian Island until Melanesians landed there and the people of Fiji are descended from both groups. I will talk more about this in the chapter on "Glucose Transporters and Human DNA. Some of the best muscles I have ever seen were on a Polynesian man from one of the smaller islands of French Polynesia, in a book I have by French writer Alain Chenevière. The man is dressed in Polynesian clothes rather than Western clothes, and he is pushing a wooden spear into a very large green fruit that doesn't look like anything you would find in the West, so it is likely that his muscles and physique were developed by just doing the things Polynesians have done for thousands of years.

I have a fir tree in my back yard. When we first bought this house back in 2003 the fir tree was small and misshapen, as though it had been hit by a bulldozer. I have never been big on killing trees, so I left the tree in to see what would happen. It was about four feet tall in those days, and is now about twenty-five feet tall, and the kink in its trunk has straightened out. For the past four years our part of Florida has had reduced rainfall, and many of the summer storms that we used to have, have disappeared. Every year I have to save the fir tree by watering it. There is a faucet near the tree in the backyard, but I walk to the front of the house and use the faucet there, which enables me to carry a watering can full of water much further. I do this because I noticed that it is a good exercise for my arms. It is worth thinking of ways you can alter normal household jobs in a way that you can use to strengthen your muscles. If you have stairs in your house, then every time you climb those stairs you strengthen the transverse abdominal muscles in your waist area. These are important muscles, if they are strong they will hold your backbone in place and protect it, if they are weak then you may get back injuries more easily. I don't have stairs in our house in Florida unfortunately, but one of the exercises I use is stair climbing. This is one of the few exercises where the more you weigh, the more calories you burn.

It is important to think about exercises you can do in your house. We all lead very busy lives, and if you have to drive somewhere it cuts into your exercise time. I am lucky in that I live in a landscaped subdivision that is beautiful to walk in. These are standard in Florida, and what this means is that I can leave my house, and as soon I am out of the front door my exercise session begins. Several years ago I went out in my car, and mapped out all the possible walking routes I can use. The longest I mapped out was nine miles, but it is possible to leave my house and walk thirty miles on paved footpaths, so for walking exercises that saves me a lot of time, and it is as good as anywhere nearby. Of course, I would far rather walk in North Carolina than in Florida, and my son and I were once stopped early in the morning on a mountain called Chimney Rock in North Carolina by two park rangers, who asked where we were from, and told us that nobody walked up the mountain, people only walked down it (you could take a bus to the top, we took the bus down instead). When they found we had driven to the area from Jacksonville the night before, a distance of 423 miles (681 kilometers), they were even more surprised.

When we arrived the heavens had opened, and it started to rain, and I had looked at my son and asked if he still wanted to hike in the rain, and he had said he was up for it. It didn't rain for that long, and we had a great time. There was a restaurant at the top of the mountain, and you could sit outside, and look down at a reservoir and a forest, which was even better. When we took the bus down the mountain, we were driven on a winding road by an old guy who had his head turned around talking to the woman in the seat in front of us. There were some huge drops, and it appeared that he didn't look at the road once, but he didn't crash so he obviously knew what he was doing. I have driven that road before in the days when private cars were allowed on it, and it is a one lane road which allowed two-way driving, and that made for quite an interesting trip up the mountain. The whole area was developed by a doctor who bought the land in the early part of the twentieth century. It is now a North Carolina State Park, and well worth a visit. My son-in-law actually proposed to my step-daughter on top of that mountain, to the accompaniment of cheers from everyone else who was on top of the mountain at the time.

Some of you may be reluctant to exercise, especially if you are not used to it. It is important to start slowly, and not go in too hard. There are a lot of tricks you can use if you are a reluctant exerciser. For example, if you are going to the gym, break the whole operation into a series of different steps, or if you like compartmentalize it. Thus getting in your car is not hard, since you do that every day. Driving to the gym is not hard, since you drive every day. Getting out of your car, and changing your clothes is something you do every day. So the actual exercise only starts when you are inside the gym, and at that point, since you are there anyway you may as well do the exercises. I work out in an unusual way in that I don't stop to rest after each set, I just work out a different set of muscles. Men in gyms who rest after each set are often going for serious muscle building, and aiming to build bulk. We are not here to do that, we are here to improve the parts of your muscles that pull sugar out of your bloodstream, and all that means is that you have to work the muscle, and not necessarily bulk it up. What we are aiming to do here is get your muscles into a situation where the GLUT 4 and GLUT 1 in your muscles (GLUTs are glucose transporters) can more easily pull sugar out of your bloodstream. There are three classes of glucose transporters, with GLUT 1 to GLUT 4 being in Class 1. GLUT 1 and GLUT 4 both respond to insulin in the bloodstream with GLUT 4 being responsible for insulin regulated glucose storage.

Glucose Transporter 1 (GLUT 1) is responsible for low level glucose intake into cells, which gives them their basic energy. Glucose transporters are important enough to this book that they share their own chapter along with human DNA, and I will go into much more detail there than I do in this chapter. Having said that, I do need to say a few things about Glucose Transporter 4 (GLUT 4) as it relates to muscle tissue.

GLUT 4 is involved in glucose transport into fat tissue (adipose tissue), and also into striated muscles (skeletal muscles and heart muscles). The heart muscle is a special type of muscle, which doesn't get tired, and has to continue working so each contraction of the heart muscle stimulates GLUT 4 to rise to the surface of the muscle cells, where it can pull in more sugar to keep the heart supplied with energy. The rest of your muscles don't have this attribute to anything like the extent of the heart muscle, so their ability to pull in sugar from the blood varies. In short, a well developed muscle will push GLUT 4 to the surface of the muscle cells, where it can pull in sugar from the blood to power the muscle. In a weak, flabby muscle GLUT 4 will not rise to the surface of the cells so easily, and two things will happen, the first thing that happens is that weak muscles will not be able to pull as much sugar out of the bloodstream as strong muscles, and the second, and more obvious thing that will happen is that weak muscles will be underpowered because they will be unable to fuel themselves efficiently.

Hopefully you see where I am going with this. As little as two weeks training can make a big difference to the ability of your muscle cells to pull in blood sugar, and that means not only will you have lower blood sugar, you will also be stronger, and will have more energy. Take hold of your right bicep (the muscle on the inside of your upper arm) with your left hand, bend your right arm at the elbow, and squeeze your right hand into a fist. Now feel that bicep, if it is super hard then well done, if it is soft or somewhere between hard and soft then there is work to be done, and it will pay huge benefits in terms of sugar sucked out of your bloodstream.

GLUT 4 was discovered by Australian cell biologist David E. James in 1988 at the age of thirty years old. The gene that encodes GLUT 4 was cloned and mapped one year later in 1989. This gene is located on Chromosome 17 on a human and Chromosome 11 on a mouse. Research into glucose transport isoforms is still ongoing, and to date thirteen glucose transporters have been identified. The function of some of the more recently discovered glucose transport isoforms is not clearly defined at present.

Our nearest relative is the chimpanzee, and the average chimpanzee can exert four times as much pressure in his or her arms as the average human. Conversely, since we walk on two legs, we can cream the chimpanzee when it comes to leg muscle strength. Walking, running, dancing and stair climbing are all exercises that can develop the legs easily. Next time you see someone in the military take a look at their legs, especially their thighs. The chances are that their thigh muscles will be much bigger than yours. Thigh muscles take time to develop, but if you can do that it pays dividends when pulling sugar out of your blood. Now before all the women reading this book tell me that they don't want huge muscles, we do not need to go that far. The muscles you will see on bodybuilders are nearly always developed using steroids. What I'm suggesting here is that you take whatever you have and make it stronger, but you do not need to bulk your muscles up. In fact, steroids can really trash your health, whether you are male or female and they are definitely not a route to go down. Also steroids will often trash your liver, and I think a lot of the tipping points into diabetes are right there in our livers, and what we are doing to them with the food we are eating now.

I have read a lot of books on weight training and bodybuilding over the years, and I have bought books by both men and women. My interest has always been in terms of fitness and keeping myself strong, rather than in competitive bodybuilding so I have been more interested in just making my muscles strong rather than bulking up. Do not, under any circumstances use a protein drink because those things are loaded with sugar, and most of the weight gain they produce is fat rather than muscle, unless you are working out for several hours each day. Just read the percentage of calories from carbohydrates and sugars on the back of a protein drink and you will be amazed, and then after that you may well be annoyed with the manufacturers. They may well work for competitive bodybuilders, but for the ordinary person looking to do what we are going to do in this book, then they are definitely not a good idea. In one of the books I read the author stated that he only knew one bodybuilder with diabetes, and I am willing to bet that was type 1 diabetes.

It is a good idea to buy a book on weight training. People often prefer to buy a book written by a member of their own sex. The best book written by a man is "The New Encyclopedia of Modern Bodybuilding" by Arnold Schwarzenegger. This is an excellent book, and the book I go to first if I want to find the right form to do a certain lift. Arnold will give you starting position, intermediate position, and ending position, which is invaluable. Any book by Robert Kennedy is also well worth adding to your collection. The best book on weight training that I have that is written by a woman is "The Eat-Clean Diet Workout" by Tosca Reno, who was married to Robert Kennedy until his death in April 2012. I want to pay tribute here to Robert Kennedy. I never met him, but his books and magazines were a great resource for me. "MuscleMag" for male readers and "Oxygen" for female readers are both great resources for anyone interested in weight training, and both these magazines were published by Robert Kennedy. Robert was the son of an Austrian father and an English mother, who were both teachers in England.

When I first began to combat high blood sugar I got up fifteen minutes earlier, and did four weight lifting exercises. These were forward wrist curls, reverse wrist curls, concentration curls, and single arm extensions. Not too many people do forward and reverse wrist curls, but I have always found them to be great exercises, and do these for a while and you will always be the person in the office who is known for his or her ability to get the top off a jar that nobody else can open. Wrist muscles often lose part of their strength after age forty, so it is good to exercise them and bring them back up to strength. It is very important to start with a small weight the first time you do forward and reverse wrist curls, as you can easily sprain your wrist. I am going to advise you to look in the weight training book you buy, as I do not have the training to advise other people (at least not in a book) how to work out with weights. Arnold Schwarzenegger and Robert Kennedy are the men for that, and Tosca Reno is the woman. I would have no problem advising someone I worked out with in a gym how to lift a weight, but for the purposes of this book then go to a proper weight training book. What I will do is tell you some of the things I do to avoid getting injured. When I first walk into a gym, I will often do the movements for the exercise without a weight in my hands. That way your tendons, ligaments, and everything else get moved without a weight pulling on them, and if they need to be stretched that is the time to do it, and not when you have a heavy weight on your arm. I will do that or perhaps I will take a five pound or ten pound weight and do the exercise, that way you are not putting full pressure on everything from the get go. The safety tips I will give you here are not exhaustive, but may help and once again rely on the trainer at the gym or on a book like Arnold Schwarzenegger's for how to lift a weight properly. Arnold is the only person who has ever told me that if my elbow aches, then I am lifting the weight with my elbow, and not with my muscle. This is important because if you lift a weight with your arm that is too heavy for the muscle, then after a few days your elbow will be very painful. For our purposes always go for a lighter weight, and not the heaviest you think you can lift because the last thing you need is to injure yourself in the first few weeks, while you are trying to drop your blood sugar. Sometimes I will do multiple sets with a weight that is lighter than I can lift, just to try and work the muscle to exhaustion. This is not something I do every time I go to the gym, but it is another way of training the muscles, and it will give them a different kind of workout. Again every time you lift a weight you are burning blood sugar, and every time your muscle burns sugar it will send out GLUT 4 receptors looking for more sugar, which will then be pulled out of your blood stream. Do that enough and you will find you are putting pressure on one of the tipping points that can tip you out of a type 2 diabetes state. Muscles are voracious eaters of sugar once you get them going, so make sure you are not the person who only exercises his or her finger on the TV remote button. There is another tipping point right there. When I was young, you had to get up and walk over to the television if you wanted to change the channel, and that at least would give you a bit of a workout. While you are standing you are using multiple muscle adjustments just to make sure you keep your balance, and the effort of lifting your body out of a chair also burns sugar. Okay, so once an hour didn't make a lot of difference, but at the same time even getting up once an hour is better than sitting there for three hours. My son is a big fan of the British show "Downton Abbey", and just before Christmas I watched a three hour marathon with him, which was a catch-up ready for the new season, which just started in January. I never sit down for three hours running, this might happen perhaps a few times a year for me, and whilst the show was very enjoyable and pulled me in, I noticed at the end of the three hours I actually felt unhealthy, and I put that down to sitting in one spot for three hours without getting up. Just walking from one end of your house to the other boosts blood circulation, and it is something you should try and do at least once an hour.

I have an excel spreadsheet which records what I did with exercising when I was climbing out of diabetes. The spreadsheet starts on November 22, 2007, which must be the first day I started exercising. I used to write the records on a sheet of paper which covered two weeks, and then transfer them and it looks as though I didn't transfer the first sheet. I was lifting weights in the morning, and either walking or stair climbing at night. The first day I have records for in terms of weight lifting, is Monday December 3, 2007, and on that day I did 300 forward wrist curls, 210 reverse wrist curls, and 120 concentration curls, which work the bicep. Although this sounds like a lot, it probably took less than fifteen minutes to do. I don't rest between reps (repetitions), I just do a different exercise instead. Typically one set of reps is eight to ten lifts. I work by doing ten reps on my right arm, and then ten reps on my left arm, and then keep switching. By the time I have done the reps for my left arm, my right arm is okay to be worked again. I will usually do 50 to 100 forward wrist curls first, and then switch to reverse wrist curls. I usually do less of those, and then I switch to either concentration curls or dumbbell curls, both of which work the bicep. I usually do two sets of ten on either arm, alternating between arms, and then I will do two sets of ten on each arm for single arm extensions, which work the triceps muscle.

Very few natural movements work the triceps muscle so this is a good one to do. That hits a good number of muscles on your arms, and if you do that for even just two weeks you will notice a big improvement. It is important to start with a weight you can handle easily, and do not be tempted to increase the weight too fast, especially as you get older as all you will do is strain yourself. Be patient and you will be rewarded, rush things and you will be jumping into the "no pain, no gain" arena, which is a waste of your time and absolutely no use to you.

It is very important to plan your routine so that you keep working. When I am doing a workout I never stop lifting. If I am not lifting, then I am putting a weight back or picking up another one. You must give weight lifting your absolute full concentration. Treat it like a job that needs to be done properly. Do not look at members of the opposite sex while you are lifting weights. It will distract you from the movement, and if you drop the weight you may injure yourself or others. You should keep talking to a minimum. Five minutes is okay, fifteen is not. Every so often you will see a person who spends an hour at the gym, but does very little actual working out, and I always wonder what they are actually doing there. Everyone occasionally will talk for a while, and if it is an occasional thing that is one thing, but if you are doing it every time you go to the gym then change your habits or you will not see any benefit.

When you first start going to a gym it will take about a month before you start to turn it into a habit, and it could well take a month before you start to enjoy it. I hated the first month I spent in a gym in America. I was there because I had to be. I had been in this country for about four months, and was working as a Cost Schedule Manager on the North Slope of Alaska, at latitude 70 degrees north in the oilfields at Prudhoe Bay. It was January, and it was dark for 24 hours a day. We flew up on January 5, 1998, and the sun didn't come up until January 19. I suspect that humans are pushed into a semi-hibernation mode in conditions like that, and one thing that happened to me was that I put on twenty pounds in one month. I worked 12 to 14 hours every day for four straight weeks until I flew back down to Anchorage, and I didn't weigh myself while I was up there. Apparently this is quite common, and young men in their twenties often put on twenty pounds in a month when they go up to the North Slope. When I realized this my immediate fear was that I would put on another twenty pounds when I flew back up six days later. I mentioned what had happened to a few of my colleagues and one of them, Mike Henderson, invited me to the gym with him and another colleague called Scott. I had already changed my diet, and switched to meat or fish plus whatever vegetables were available as long as they weren't cooked in any kind of sauce or butter. Mike was a very formative influence on me, and set many really good exercise habits in place both for me and for Scott. Scott's last name was Brower, and if anyone who reads this book in Anchorage, Alaska knows Mike or Scott then please give them my email address (at the back of the book), and tell them I would love to hear from them.

When I started exercising with Mike and Scott, Mike was 48, I was 38, and Scott was 28. I had been in very good shape in England, but moving to Alaska had already had effects on my fitness. In England I ran on the spot every night, but my new wife kept her house extremely hot, and it was just too hot to run on the spot in the house. Once October hit, it was just too cold to go outside and exercise. If I went up to Alaska now I would just learn cross country skiing, and go on the trails up there because that is a great exercise, and also very strenuous but I didn't know that then.

Mike was ten years older than me and twenty years older than Scott, but he was actually in better shape than both of us put together. Mike and Scott helped get me through those first thirty days of working out. At the time I was working out solely because I knew I had to, or I might put another twenty pounds on, and some days I had to force myself to go to the gym with them. Going to the gym or lifting weights is never a problem these days, and I always enjoy it. Sometimes I don't do it as often as I should, but I never, ever sit in a gym or on a weight bench, and wonder why I am there. These days it is always a pleasure to work out, and Mike Henderson has to take a good part of the credit for getting me into the situation where I took pleasure in working out. Mike used a mixture of teasing and encouragement, and he made the whole experience of working out fun. He was incredibly fit and had been working out for years, and he taught me a lot. The work season for pipeline construction on the North Slope lasted from January to April, while the ground was frozen, and the three of us worked out pretty much every day in the gym. Over the first thirty days of working out, I lost the entire twenty pounds that I had put on, and when the construction season ended, I was in pretty good shape. I was moved to another part of the company the following year, and I lost touch with Scott and Mike when I moved to a different company after a lot of production was shut down on the North Slope after BP bought ARCO.

I lived in Alaska for four years, and the exercise habits I picked up from Mike and Scott stuck. Most of the time I lived up there I worked out in gyms. I went to a small back street gym run by an ex-military man in Wasilla, where we lived for a while. I don't remember the name of that gym, but it was a great place to work out. All the equipment was second hand, but I learnt a lot there. Sometime around then I picked up "The New Encyclopedia of Modern Bodybuilding" by Arnold Schwarzenegger, and I started working out in Gold's Gym in Anchorage. This was a great place to work out, and I used to go there at lunchtime a lot, and also on Fridays after work.

It is important to select your gym carefully. You are there to work out, and sometimes the gym with a spa, and the best advertising is not the best place for you. If the gym is crowded, and there are too many people around when you are trying to work out, that can be a problem. Gyms with second hand equipment, and not too many clients can often be great places to work out because you can often get on all the machines. When I am at the gym, every moment I am waiting to use a machine is wasted time. If that happens I will often go and use another machine, but I really need to be able to get on most of the things I want to get on first time, so make sure you don't end up in a gym where you have to wait a lot. If all the gyms in your area tend to be busy, then find a time to go when they are not busy. Be flexible too, and you will often be lifting iron while other people are standing around, which means you will get more from your workout than they will from theirs. If you are lifting weights, then give the weights your absolute full attention, and do not get distracted, either by a conversation or by looking at a member of the opposite sex. Never lift a weight while you are in the middle of a conversation, that is a really good way to injure yourself.

It is also well worth having a small gym at home (or a large one if you are lucky enough to have the space). My wife recently reorganized all the gym equipment in the house into my step-daughter's old bedroom. My wife really wanted to put all the gym equipment in the garage, but it is 95 degrees or higher in there most of the summer so we managed to talk her out of it. I bought a weight bench and a lot of barbells from the son of a couple we bought a house from in Alaska, and I have added a lot of weights over the years. If I walk into the weight room, the first thing I see on the left is a Reebok stepper, which is actually very useful. This cost me $20 to $30, and you can set a variable height to make a step up, step down piece of equipment. This works the calves, front of the thighs, and probably the back of the thighs as well. It also works the transverse abdominal muscles below your abdominal muscles so it is a great piece of equipment. I have said before that it is well worth your while to have strong transverse abdominal muscles, as they will help hold your backbone in place and prevent injury to it. Behind the stepper is a weight bench. I use that for bench presses, and also to sit on for forward and reverse wrist curls. If there is an exercise that can be done standing up or sitting down, then I will usually do it standing up, as my belief is that you can keep your back straight more easily if you are standing than sitting down. I bought my weight bench twelve years ago, and it was second hand so I don't know how old it is. I have taken good care of it and it is still going strong. With many things you can buy them, and never need to replace them as they are made to be strong. Everything in my gym was made in America though, I don't know about stuff made abroad that has been made cheaply, so be careful with that. I would certainly buy American for weight equipment because you can't afford to have something break on you when you have a heavy weight in your hands. Make sure that it is actually made in the United States, and that it does not just have an American manufacturer's name on it.

Next to the weight bench is a treadmill that I bought for my wife when we lived in Alaska. I have used the treadmill on occasions, but I prefer to walk outside. Treadmills have their place though, one of the trainers at Gold's Gym in Alaska who was incredibly well muscled used to do forty minutes a day on the treadmill with the incline set at maximum. The treadmill faces the corner of the room, and the two windows face out over a lake with a fir tree to one side in our backyard, which is a nice view. This is the same fir tree that I have had to save every year for the last four years, due to our now weird weather, and I am looking forward to the time these unusual droughts stop, and the regular rains get going again. Our weather is almost backwards now, and it rained again heavily today even though January is supposed to be a dry month in Jacksonville. We can always tell when it is going to rain, as the dog's face changes due to the fact that she is scared of thunderstorms, and we often refer to the "doggy barometer" in our house. She usually knows that it is going to rain half an hour to an hour before it actually happens.

The other piece of equipment we have in the exercise room is an ab-lounger. This originally belonged to my step-daughter, and my son uses it now. I just look at him on it, and imagine what someone over forty could strain doing those movements so I will never go on it. He likes it, and we even went out and bought another one when the first one broke. Now that I think about it, the ab-lounge looks too flimsy to have been made in America, and this perfectly illustrates my point earlier as you would not want to be doing one of the extreme movements you do on that, and have it break under you. I suspect from the weight of the thing that the bars holding it together are hollow, or they are not made of steel, and that is just wrong in my opinion. Like I said earlier, be careful what you buy.

The other items we have in the room hold weights. One is a Gold Gym weight holder, and it holds twelve barbells in two rows. We also have another weight holder that holds eight barbells. These are really strong, and they are also built to be stable, which is vital with something holding that much weight. They are the same design that you will see in professional gyms, although the ones in gyms usually hold a lot more weights than mine do. The weights I have in the room vary from ten pounds to thirty-five pounds. I may have a couple of forty pound weights, but they are in my son's room as he tends to lift heavier weights than I do. The only other thing in the room is a picture of two Bengal tigers that my step-daughter left when she moved out It is a nice picture, in that the mother tiger has white fur with tiger markings and the cub has normal tiger coloring. If you look at a tiger's face, one of the interesting things is that the tiger, the lion and the domestic cat seem to have exactly the same shape in the way their noses are shaped, which seems quite unusual given their different sizes.

Before we leave the weight lifting section, I just want to let you know which exercises I was doing, and how many of those I did in a week. Like I said earlier, I started doing weight lifting in late November 2007, and by February 2008 I was lifting weights in the morning before going to work, and going to the gym at lunchtime. I aimed to work out five days a week and leave the weekends free, and I pretty much stuck to that, although nowadays I use Saturday as a catch up day if anything happens to interrupt my exercise schedule. Bear in mind that I did a lot more exercises in those first eight weeks than I probably do now, and that is important. You don't have to do this at the rate I did it forever. First you must drain your sugar reservoirs, and that will put pressure on one of the tipping points. Once you have exerted enough pressure, you will flip your body out of type 2 diabetes, and at that point you can maintain this state with less exercise and less dietary control. If you are a woman and you feel you are building muscles, and you don't like that, then stop working out so hard and they will fade within a month. Having said that, working out without using steroids is unlikely to produce huge muscles. I remember when I was doing my accounting degree, we had one guy on the course who worked out for six hours a day. He drank six pints of milk a day and ate a lot of protein, but he didn't use steroids, and he looked nothing like the muscle bound men of today. He was incredibly strong, I once saw him pick up another guy on the course as though he was as light as a feather. He just put his hands on the other guy's hips and hoisted him up to six feet in the air in an instant, and he made it look effortless.

The exercises I did in a week once I was up to speed are as follows, and this is based on fifteen minutes of exercise in the morning plus a lunch time session at the gym. In week ended February 17, 2008, I did 1,450 forward wrist curls, 800 reverse wrist curls, 390 single arm extensions working the triceps muscle, 240 bench presses, 340 dumbbell curls working the biceps, and 290 lat machine pull downs. I also probably used the machines that worked my arms in the gym too, although I don't have those recorded so it might be that I hadn't started doing that yet. Where it says 340 dumbbell curls then this means both arms, so each arm was worked 340 times. Doing all that in one week will strengthen your muscles a lot. This is just one muscle working, imagine how much GLUT 4 was activated in just that one muscle in just one week, and imagine how much sugar was pulled out of my blood stream just to work that one muscle. Muscle burns far more calories per hour than fat too, which means your sugar reservoirs are drained much faster if you have muscles. Although those numbers look like a lot, they are not. I can do 100 forward wrist curls fairly quickly. I start with 20 on each arm, and then do 10 alternating between arms. If you use my method of always keeping lifting something, things will go much quicker. This requires balance and thought, but once you have the hang of it then it is pretty easy. Like I said earlier, if I wanted to build bulk then this would not be the best way to lift iron, but you are working your muscles to burn sugar and activate your glucose transporters.

I just looked at my blood sugar records, which are on a separate spreadsheet, and week ending February 17, 2008 was the last time I had a blood sugar reading over 126 mg/dl (7.0 mmol/L), and that was on the morning of Tuesday February 12, 2008 at 6:25am and was 130 mg/dl (7.22 mmol/L), which was only just over. Now, this illustrates the value of keeping good records, because I can look back almost five years later, and say that when I pulled myself out of diabetes the last bad blood sugar reading was on Tuesday February 12, 2008 at 6:25am and was 130 mg/dl (7.22 mmol/L). In fact, after writing the chapter on "Climbing out of Diabetes", I found that I only had two blood sugar readings over 126 mg/dl (7.0 mmol/L) after Sunday January 6, 2008, and these were both marginally over, so I was pretty much done with type 2 diabetes by January 7, 2008. There is much more detail about this in the chapter on "Climbing out of Diabetes", and in Appendix 1 so I will not go over it again here.

The morning blood sugar readings are always the hardest to clear, and I have written more about the readings in the section called "Climbing out of Type 2 Diabetes" and in Appendix 1, but this gives you a feel for how quickly a quietly determined man can clear his blood sugar reservoirs to a point where he flips himself out of diabetes. Of course, a quietly determined woman can do exactly the same thing, but since I am a man living in a man's body I have no idea what it is like to live in a woman's body. However, what works for one sex often works for the other. The important point to note here is that I am just an ordinary man, and if I can do it then you can do it. Weight lifting was not my only exercise, but I know that I did ease back once I had the situation under control. This whole book is just about draining your blood sugar reservoirs, and as long as you keep them low, and well away from being full then you have control, and if you have control you can live a normal life. To a large extent being a little overweight and having to exercise is of great benefit because if you are thin and never work out in your life, then you may be less fit and die earlier than somebody was forced to exercise and look after himself or herself.

So to recap let's talk about a battle situation again. Remember that type 2 diabetes is your enemy, and you have to treat him as such. In the UK, they don't have the Highland Games in England, only in Scotland, and having grown up in England I had never been to a Highland Games until I came to America. I went to the Highland Games in Eagle River, Alaska the summer after I came to America, and I watched a talk by a Scottish American about the weapons used by the Scots when they went into battle. The Scots had a sword, a knife, and a fearsome weapon called a dirk, which is as long as a man's forearm and they used all three very quickly when they went into the attack, and God help you if you were on the receiving end. Weight lifting is an incredible weapon in your arsenal because of the effect it has on the GLUT 4 in your muscles, and the changes it makes to the ability of GLUT 4 to pull sugar out of your blood stream. If you meet type 2 diabetes on the battlefield with the weapon of weight lifting, then you can drive in the dirk and gut him. You will not kill him with that, and he can fight on, but you will have changed the course of the battle, and once you have gutted him then you will win and he will lose, and it is only a matter of time until that happens so make absolutely sure that weight lifting is in your arsenal of weapons when you go into battle with type 2 diabetes.

In the next two sections I will talk about walking, which is something anybody can do, and then we'll look at heavy exercises such as running, stair climbing, bike riding, and the like. After that,

I want to look at Tai Chi and yoga, both of which can build stamina and muscle.

Humans are built to walk. Compared with many other mammals we have incredible stamina. That was our one strength in a world where many other animals were stronger, and faster than we were. Consider this, one million years ago a chimpanzee could sit on the branch of a tree a mere fifteen feet from a lion, and be perfectly safe. A human ancestor, on the other hand who found himself fifteen feet from a lion rapidly became dinner. We may only be here now due to the ability of our ancestors to follow prey for hours, or days, until they wore it out. Persistence is a survival trait, and early hunters needed to have it if they were to eat. We are essentially a primate that found itself out of its element when the climate changed, and there were no longer trees to support the primate that split into us and the chimpanzees. The ancestors of the chimpanzees kept the trees, and our ancestors were left to forage as best they could on the ground. The result of that was to turn us into a creature that could walk long distances. There is much more food in a tropical rainforest environment than in a savannah environment. The Earth's axis moves over long periods of time, and the latitude for the tropics varies between 21 degrees and 24 degrees. When the axis is in the right place, Africa has a monsoon just the same as India, but that monsoon is dependent on heat rising and sucking in air from the Indian Ocean, and it can only operate when the Earth's axis is in the right position to heat the right area of land in Africa. We are a species which has grown up under conditions where the climate jumped backwards and forwards, and one of the reasons we are still here was our ancestors' ability to walk out of a bad area, and into an area where there was more food. There are settlements in Africa right now where it is dry now, but even five hundred years ago the land was covered in trees. Now that we have permanent settlements many people live in areas that they would have once walked right out of.

When I was in my twenties, I used to work in an office with a woman who did a lot of marathons. She told me one day about how she had done a cross country walking marathon the year before. She was a big fan of Labrador dogs, and she told me that if you bought a Labrador you had to be prepared to walk it every day because they were a dog that needed to be walked a lot. She took her two year old Labrador on the cross country marathon and wore it out. She said the dog was fine for the first eighteen miles, but after that it became tired, whereas she was still able to carry on. The dog was young and finished the marathon with her, but this gives an interesting comparison of just how far we are able to walk, and how we are able to out walk other mammals.

Walking is one of the easiest ways to lower the levels of sugar stored in your blood sugar reservoirs. Almost everybody can walk, and even if you are not used to walking you can very quickly get up to decent distances. My feeling is that you have to walk at least forty minutes, before you really begin to impact your blood sugar reservoirs. If I walk five miles it may take an hour and a half, and I know I have done a good walk, but if I walk two miles it doesn't feel as though it had the same effect. When I was in my thirties I would often go out on my own, and hike along an old railway track that had been torn up and resurfaced as a hiking trail. The line was closed back in 1962, in the infamous Beeching railway cuts that chopped many branch lines out of the UK's rail network. The rails were worth money as scrap so they were torn up and melted down. Twenty years later, many of the old lines were resurfaced as hiking trails. It rains so much in the UK that a track like that would have been a sea of mud if it was not resurfaced and drained properly, and I have walked some of the tracks many times in the rain. There was one old rail track I used to walk quite often that followed the A515 road between Alsop en le Dale and Buxton. At the time I lived in a place called Sawley between the cities of Nottingham and Derby, and starting early on a Saturday or Sunday I could be at the trailhead within forty minutes of leaving my house. People born in Scotland are hard wired for cold weather, and I have walked that trail in winter, spring, and fall, but never in summer. In winter it is cold enough so that you have to keep moving, or you get cold no matter how well wrapped up you are. I remember one great walk where I walked for six and a half hours with two fifteen minute stops for sandwiches. As long as I was moving I was warm, but as soon as I stopped the cold began to creep in. In winter in England I didn't even need gloves, as after fifteen minutes of walking the blood circulation in my hands would increase to the point that they kept warm. In those days I never had to worry about blood sugar levels. That may have been because I was younger or it may have been because I routinely did long walks, and I also ran on the spot in my house every night for forty minutes. One girlfriend I had when I was thirty-three was following behind me on a narrow trail in Greece when she told me that I had the biggest calves she had ever seen on a man. I weighed just 175 pounds at the time (79 kilos), and my calves were well developed because I ran on the spot so much.

Let's look at walking and see what you can do there. If you do walk already then that is great, add it to your arsenal of weapons against type 2 diabetes. If you have not exercised for years, and some of you will be in this position, then walking is a safe way to start. You should always see your doctor before starting any kind of exercise routine, even walking, so make sure that you do that. If you have type 2 diabetes and you are taking any kind of medications for blood sugar control such as insulin or glucophage drugs then hypoglycemia (extremely low blood sugar) can occur and you should never change your exercise or diet routine before having a serious discussion with your doctor first. Please see the warning at the beginning of the book.

If you are not used to walking, then don't go in hard, just try half a mile or a mile to start with, and be careful with temperatures if you are older. If you have any kind of heart condition, take someone with you. If you don't exercise, you will find even walking hard at first. Make sure you have good shoes. I use either New Balance or Nike. New Balance recently shortened the length of the laces on their sneakers from 60 inches to 53 inches, which makes it hard to double knot them. I have not written to New Balance yet about this, but I bought Nike after they did this as you really need to be able to double knot a shoelace to stop it from untying itself on a hike. This is cost cutting gone mad because the laces have to make up less than 1% of the cost of the shoe, and New Balance just turned off a customer who usually buys at least four sets of sneakers a year. I recently bought two sets of Nikes, one pair was made in Indonesia, and one pair was made in China. I found that the ones made in Indonesia fit me really well, but the ones made in China pull at my toenails and are not as good. I also had the same problem when New Balance switched their production to China, although I think they are back to making them in America now.

If your thighs rub together, then use some kind of lotion. Most men don't want to do this, but if you chafe your thighs then you will not be walking after a few days. My son and I recently did the Jacksonville 15 kilometer walk, and all the medical stations were advising people to use Vaseline, or some kind of lotion on any areas that chafed. Obviously if you buy new shoes then break them in, and don't do a long hike in them. I just use sneakers for walking on a normal sidewalk, but if you are hiking in the country use proper walking boots. I have a really good example of the need to always have hiking boots. Back in 2007 my sister remarried in England, and I arranged to meet my old hiking friend, Dave, for two days hiking. My son, Nathan, was old enough to do a proper hike by then so he came along too. We stood in the parking lot about to start the hike, and I was joking with Nathan that in many of the walks Dave and I had done there was always an incredibly hard bit that lasted about an hour, and that is true. I have walked along cliff tops in Wales with seventy foot drops below, hanging on to grass in high winds to stop from being blown off. I have run along a beach made entirely of large stones, and trusted Dave when he said that as long as we kept running fast, the stones would take our weight without tipping. He was right, but when I look back on that time one of us could have easily broken an ankle that day. I have walked along rocks in Wales that had been turned as smooth as glass by river water, alongside signs warning us not to do that, Dave wanted to do it anyway, and there was no other way up the river so we just had to be careful and hope we didn't fly off the edge, but the view at the end of the walk was well worth it.

Nathan laughed when I told him some of the things that Dave had done, especially the one about the cliff top walks. I said to Nathan that now we were both older, and in our forties there wouldn't be anything like that anymore. Well, within twenty minutes we were climbing up a path which was incredibly steep, but which would no problem in normal weather. However, it had rained continuously for a week, and the path was an ocean of mud, and very slippery. Nathan had come with boots from the United States, but my British walking boots had cracked in Alaska (they are not designed for minus 20 fahrenheit), so I had needed to buy some more. I almost didn't buy them, and we had made a special detour the day before just to buy some boots, but if I hadn't bought those boots I would have slid right off that hillside as it was so slippery. Dave and I are both experienced hikers, and we both knew how to brace ourselves on the slope by putting our feet at a sideways angle, which greatly increases the force you are exerting on the ground, giving you better traction. Nathan did not know how to do this and he slipped, and grabbed a thorn bush trying to save himself. I looked back, and realized that he could fall two hundred feet so I went behind him and told him to stay in the middle. I also told him how to brace himself and said that if he slipped, I would dive on top of him and break his fall as I was really worried he would end up sliding all the way down the trail. I knew a British woman who fell like that once, and although she wasn't badly hurt, she ended quite badly bruised from bouncing off trees on the way down which was no fun. We made it to the top without any major problems, but Nathan was a bit annoyed that we had subjected him to that. He told me later on that he had considered throwing both me and Dave off the top of the ridge. I had always thought Nathan was serious about that and Dave was a bit alarmed when I told him, but Nathan told me just a couple of days ago that he was joking at the time. I said all that just to give you an example of how different that hike could have been if I hadn't stopped to buy boots, so always be prepared and take the right footwear.

You will also need to have what I call have a heavy exercise in your arsenal, something that will rip the sugar right out of your body. This might be running, it might be stair climbing, cross country skiing, or some other exercise. Even something like cutting down trees burns an incredible amount of energy, and I know that some Americans are into doing that. I used to run regularly when I was in my twenties, but I injured my knee running on concrete in the wrong kind of footwear when I was twenty-six years old, and I have never been able to run on concrete since, even in running shoes. The first run is always okay, but when I get up the next day, my knee is fine until I try and walk downstairs, and then it feels like somebody is sliding a knife blade into the side of my knee. At the time I did this, I had friends who had gone under the knife and had knee surgery, and none of them were happy with the results so I didn't do anything about it. It has never bothered me since unless I run on concrete, and I can still run on the spot, so I did a lot of that in my twenties and thirties. When I went to Alaska, as I said earlier my wife kept her house far too hot, and so I had to give up running on the spot. I have never really gotten back into it properly, and that was a great exercise that I used to do in England for forty minutes each night. Had I kept that up I suspect I would never have gotten high blood sugar, and I have tried to get back into it but haven't been able to do it properly. That is a classic case of "use it or lose it" so never give up on an exercise, especially as you get older. You can do just about anything in your twenties and thirties, but once you hit your forties you need to keep active.

When I used to drive to work in Anchorage, Alaska I would drive down 5th Avenue before turning south on C Street, and I would see a lot of tourists walking. Many were elderly people, and it would always surprise me how much trouble some of them had walking. I think part of the problem was the climate in those days as there was snow on the ground for long periods in the northern states in winter, which meant people had to drive everywhere. One of the advantages in England was that there was often very little parking, so if you worked in a town or city it was often easier to walk into the town at lunchtime rather than try and take your car in. Some people may not see this as an advantage, but I did at the time.

If I had my choice I would probably run five miles a day or maybe even more, and that is a good one to try if it suits you. My personal heavy exercise of choice is stair climbing. I got into this when I worked inside the Beltway in Washington D.C. and we lived in an apartment for a while. I used to walk up and down two flights of stairs. I originally started doing this as my job was very stressful at the time. I was moved to a different section where three of us worked on one job. The woman who was working on it warned me that the boss was planning to make me do the whole thing on my own. I could see that she was right, but there was nothing I could do about it. I streamlined it as much as I could when I had the whole lot handed to me, and I was able to manage the whole thing in a month, but it was quite a stressful job so I started stair climbing just to cope with the stress. The alternative was probably alcohol or some kind of tablets, and there was no way I was doing either of those. I started slowly because I had not climbed many stairs in the last year, but once I got into it I climbed fifty flights of stairs every night five days a week. I got to know just about all my neighbors in our set of apartments, and I had many great conversations with them as it was surprising how many people were interested in what I was doing. My calves and the transverse abdominal muscles in my abdomen both became rock hard, and I was extremely fit at the time. If you can do this then it is a great exercise, but be very careful, and I will give you a triple health warning on that one. Do not even think about doing this without talking to your doctor first, and if you do try it then make sure you take plenty of breaks. I am a strong man with plenty of stamina, but I will guarantee that if you are able to do this then it will take most of the stress of American life away. I am referring to the work lives we have to live in this country when I say this, you may be lucky and not have a stressful job, but most of the people I know have stressful jobs. I once sat in a truck with a Canadian woman on the North Slope of Alaska, and she made the comment that all the Americans on the North Slope worked far too hard with too little regard for their health. I was new to America at the time, so I really couldn't comment on that, but I think one of our problems over here is that many people have to work too hard with too little time to recoup their energies. I worked with a man in Washington D.C. who told me he hadn't had a day off for three years. I happened to know that they were paying him $150,000 a year, which meant that they had paid him $450,000 in the last three years, and it was on the tip of my tongue to tell him that if he bought a machine that cost $450,000, and then ran it without any kind of maintenance then it would almost certainly break down. I didn't say anything because you never know how something like that will be received, but a few months after that he developed type 2 diabetes. He was a good guy, and I still think about him from time to time. At the time type 2 diabetes was not as common as it is now, and we were all shocked that he had gotten it. I was pretty much the same age as him and it certainly shocked me, and most of the people we worked with were in their forties too. He had fallen into the same trap I fell into a few years later in Florida though, he was working too many hours, and probably didn't have time to exercise. I remember when we worked in that office, we had a few month ends where we worked until 4 am. I remember driving home at 4 am one night in the snow, grabbing about two hours sleep, and getting up again and going back in the next morning. Of course, if you do that you do nothing useful the next day, but at least you are there, which is really what is important at the time. I am not complaining by the way, I have always been well paid for doing this, but it can wreak havoc on your body if you are not careful. If you do have a job like this that is well paid but hard on your body, then always make sure you save the extra money you are paid and do not fritter it away.

There is a line from the film "No Country for Old Men", where Tommy Lee Jones says "This country is hard on its people", referring to America and that is certainly true. Having said that, I would not want to live anywhere else. I have been given chances in America that I would never have been given in England, and as long as you are prepared to work hard there is no limit to what you can do in America. When I walk through airports, or fairs, or other places where there are lots of Americans, I feel like I am walking with my brothers and sisters, and I didn't feel like that in England. Perhaps I would have felt like that if I had grown up in Scotland, instead of in England, because there is a difference between the English and the Scots. When I read a book by the Scottish author, Ian Rankin, called "Rebus's Scotland" when he described the Scottish character I could see myself in there. I once worked for an English company with a branch in Glasgow, and when the person in charge of the Glasgow office came down, he asked me where in Scotland I was from. When I asked him how he knew I was from Scotland since I have an English accent, he told me that he could tell from my face that I was from north of the border.

I have an excellent book on running by the Japanese author, Haruki Murakami, called "What I Talk About When I Talk About Running". Haruki Murakami is the only author besides J.K. Rowling, who has his books issued on the same day all over the world. When I read an article about this, Murakami had just issued a book called "1Q84" set in two parallel worlds. I bought it because I am fascinated by stories like that, and when I read it I noticed that the book was written at a very high intellectual level. After I read that book I bought more of Murakami's books, and I bought his book on running because I wanted to find out more about the man. It is always fascinating to read a book by a person from a totally different culture than yours. The world is a better place because we are all so different, and you learn far more by reading a book written by a man or woman who speaks a different language than you do than if you read a book written by an author from your own country. One thing that struck me when I read Murakami's book on running was how important exercise was to him, and also how much drive he had. A lot of reviews on the book are from people who didn't necessarily like the book, but I think that you can get a lot from it, and it is well worth looking at with a view to buying. It is a while since I read the book now, but one thing I liked was how exercise permeated the writer's whole life, and how important it was for him that he exercised. If you are embarking on a lifetime of exercise, which I hope you are if you read this book and want to free yourself from type 2 diabetes, then Murakami's book on running may be very valuable to you even if you are not a runner.

I am fascinated by the Japanese and by Japan in general. I have two books written by a British man called Alan Booth, who went to Japan in his early twenties. His book "The Roads to Sata: A 2000-Mile Walk Through Japan" is a fascinating account of walking from one end of Japan to the other. Booth was fluent in both spoken and written Japanese, and he walked through the back roads of Japan staying in ryokans, which are a type of Japanese inn. This is a fascinating book, and one I have read several times, each time getting something more from it.

I mentioned these two books because both authors have a kind of quiet determination about them to finish what they started, and there are subtle messages in both books that can enter your subconscious and help you with your determination to exercise. You cannot beat type 2 diabetes without having exercise in your life. Like I have said several times in this book, you must attack like the Russian army of the Czars from several different directions at once, and exercise is vital. On days that I cannot exercise for one reason or another I sometimes do not know what to do with myself, as exercise is now so ingrained in my way of life. In his book "The New Encyclopedia of Modern Bodybuilding" Arnold Schwarzenegger talks about always doing some kind of exercise when he stays in hotel rooms, and there is a lot to be said for that philosophy. We were never made to sit around and lounge in chairs, and that is one reason why people who spend their days like that end up so unhealthy.

It is very important to have an exercise routine and stick to it. My routine of five days a week, with the weekends off, works well for me. I don't think you can do any less than this during the first eight weeks while you're bringing your blood sugar down. After that, you may be able to pull back a bit. I have always enjoyed exercise, so I have just stayed with doing it five days a week. It is very easy to slip, and you must guard against this. One way I did that, was to enter all my exercise records into an excel spreadsheet. If you do this then you can do a month by month comparison. If you buy this book, and are not familiar with using excel, but you have excel on your computer, then email me at the email address at the back of this book and I will be happy to send you a copy of my exercise spreadsheet. I will leave my own numbers in so that you can see how the report is set up, and I will add blank sheets that you can use yourself. Once I had several months of exercises under my belt I would do comparisons with monthly totals, and if anything had changed I could quickly see it. Some months I might walk twenty miles less than other months, and it is always good to see that. The sooner you know about something like that, the sooner you can correct it.

I am not a believer in just doing more and more exercise. If you do that then sooner or later your subconscious will rebel, and you will find that you just stop doing exercises completely and that is not a good idea. I have studied hypnosis a lot, and when I was in my mid twenties I spent a lot of time experimenting with self-hypnosis, which is where you give yourself mental commands and attempt to hypnotize yourself by going in through the parasympathetic nervous system. This is actually quite difficult because you have to keep one part of your mind aware, while hypnotizing the other part, but with practice it is perfectly possible. I was able to get into quite deep trances doing this, and one side effect of this was to break down some of the barriers between the conscious mind, and the subconscious mind. This can be quite useful because your subconscious mind is often aware that something is wrong well before the conscious mind. Often your subconscious mind will try and alert you when you have forgotten something, such as an important file or your keys, but most people do not hear the message. Your subconscious mind can also tell you if you are about to injure yourself, for example, if you are straining a muscle, and if you can train yourself to listen to your subconscious this can be quite valuable.

I have read all kinds of interesting articles about hypnosis, some of which are quite surprising. Sometimes hypnotists do stupid things, and I read about one case in a laboratory experiment where a subject was hypnotized not to feel pain, at which point the experimenter began to jab him in the back of the hand with a sharp needle. Now, once or twice should be enough to demonstrate that this works, but in this case the experimenter kept jabbing the subject. After repeatedly doing this, another part of the subject's mind came to the surface and informed the experimenter that although the conscious mind could not feel the pain, it could, and it informed him that he needed to stop. The hypnotist was so astonished, that he stopped immediately.

I have many interesting examples from my experiences with breaking down the barrier between the conscious, and subconscious mind. In a crisis situation, I have always sprung straight into action. What happens in this kind of situation is that a part of your subconscious takes over. It can think faster than you can, it can move faster than you can, and it does not make mistakes. In one of these situations, I once ran down a steep flight of stairs, taking the stairs three at a time because I needed to get to a phone as fast as possible to call an ambulance for my first wife because I thought that she was seriously ill (I was wrong, it was worse than that). I was only thirty years old at the time, and although I was fit and strong, there is no way I could have taken stairs three at a time without ending up crashing to the bottom of the stairs. Going down the stairs was like being a passenger in my own head, I knew where my feet were going to go but they were placed with far more accuracy than my conscious mind could have done it. British stairs are much narrower than American stairs, and people fall down flights of stairs much more often in Britain than they do in America.

There was another time a few years later when I was on a large tourist boat sailing from the Greek island of Corfu to the islands of Paxos and Antipaxos. Paxos is bigger than Antipaxos, and that was where we were going to have lunch, but we went right by there and anchored in a secluded bay off the coast of Antipaxos. It was a beautiful scene, and they announced that anyone who wanted to dive off the boat into the water could do so. Within a minute or two one person had gone as high as he could on the boat, and he jumped at least thirty feet (ten meters) into the water. I hadn't jumped off a diving board since I was at school when I was fifteen years old so I decided to do the intermediate one, which was about twenty feet high. There was a line, so I waited in turn, watching other people jump off and watching others just go into the ocean from the edge of the deck rather than diving. When it was my turn I jumped. I had decided to just jump into the water, and hit feet first rather than diving. The interesting thing was that as soon as I jumped into space, I felt something in the back of my head suddenly wake up. This was fascinating because it was the same part of my mind that springs into action when a crisis situation unfolds. I had the impression that it had just been dozing in the back of my head, and not really paying attention. The interesting thing was that it thought I had done something really stupid and that we were going to die. It was fascinating to feel my subconscious come up to full power inside my head and examine all possible options. Time slowed down, and it felt to me almost as though it took five to ten minutes to hit the water, even though it must have only been seconds. Somewhere during the drop my subconscious realized that it was not going to die, and then it went quiescent again, and I hit the water with a feeling of exhilaration.

I think that is pretty much it for exercise. If you want to free yourself from type 2 diabetes, you will have to exercise, and it is one of the main prongs in your attack. Walking is a powerful tool, and has the added benefit of keeping the circulation in your legs in good shape if you do it regularly. Muscles that are well worked have a better blood supply than those that don't, which is always a good thing if you have diabetes. Use a heavy exercise as well if you can, depending on your age and ability, and also use weights.

Weight lifting with free weights, and with machines, has the advantage that you can set the weight to suit yourself and you can often get a lot of benefits with even quite light weights.

In the next section I am going to look at yoga and Tai Chi, which are a different kind of exercise, but are well worth trying.

Yoga, Tai Chi and the Five Tibetans

<u>Important Warning on Hypoglycemia (abnormally low blood sugar) for Persons Taking Insulin, Glucophage Drugs or any other Medications to Control Blood Sugar Levels</u>

Please read the warning at the start of this book. The exercise methods and dietary methods used in this book are capable of causing significant drops in blood sugar levels. Any person reading this book who is on any kind of medication to control blood sugar must talk to his or her physician before trying any of the exercise methods or dietary methods used in this book. If you are taking any medication, do not make dietary changes or exercise changes without the assistance of a physician, as medication adjustment will be necessary to prevent excessive lowering of the blood sugar level (hypoglycemia). Hypoglycemia from using too much medication can be dangerous. Please make sure your physician reads through Appendix 1 carefully so that he or she can make note of potential large blood sugar changes in very short time periods. If you are on medication to control blood sugar I would very strongly suggest that you make walking your main exercise to reduce blood sugar levels, and that you be very careful with other forms of exercise.

I put yoga and Tai Chi into a separate section on their own. I was originally going to just roll them into the exercise section, but they are different from the normal exercises done by Westerners. One of the reasons I put them into a separate section is because both techniques claim to be able to affect the energy fields running through the human body. Western science can't see these energy fields, and it can't measure them, so Western science says that they can't be there. I don't believe that, and I think this is another area that needs serious study. I said earlier that in Soviet times, two Russian scientists were able to diagnose illnesses by using a galvanometer to measure the electrical fields at the acupuncture points. How hard would it be for us to try and duplicate this? A seventeen year old schoolboy could probably have a go at this in his school science lab, and yet Western scientists won't touch something like this for fear of ruining their reputations. It will hold us back in the West if we are not prepared to be open-minded.

It may be that the whole electrical field theory inside the body is garbage, but what if it is not? What if a simple realignment of energy fields could cure some of our major diseases? I have heard of many cases where someone has been told that he or she will never walk again without crutches, and after a year of yoga they are more flexible than many people without back injuries. Surely we should be swarming all over this and investigating it. At the same time, we should not blindly accept everything we are told about yoga, or energy fields without investigating it. I am fairly open-minded, and that has allowed me to achieve many things that would be otherwise closed to me. For example, if I take a piece of string with a small weight on the end, set it to approximately 31.5 inches in length, and hold it over a piece of steel such as an ordinary kitchen knife, then my autonomous nervous system will make small muscles in my wrist vibrate to a defined pattern. I have no conscious control over those muscles, and this will only work if the string is set to exactly the right length, but it will vibrate a certain number of times and then stop. It will then repeat the cycle. I could do the same thing with copper, or gold, or another element, but I would have to use a different length of string. I read how to do this once in a book written by a British Army major, and it took me ten minutes to cut a small piece of wood for a weight and tie it onto the string, and then make it work.

Western science cannot explain why this happens. To a casual observer it appears that the string moves by itself, but that is not the case. The string is moved by rhythmic movements of the small muscles in my wrist. That can be measured by science, but what cannot be measured, or understood by Western science, is why my wrist muscles only vibrate for steel (the element iron) at a string length of approximately 31.5 inches, for copper at a different length, and for gold at a different length. If I set the string to 31 inches, or 32 inches, then absolutely nothing happens and the muscles in my wrist stay still, but somewhere in between at approximately 31.5 inches, the muscles in my wrist suddenly start vibrating. I say this just to let you know that there are some real anomalies in our world. Back in the 1960s the BBC checked this out with an archaeologist called Tom Lethbridge, and Lethbridge said in his book that the BBC sound engineer told him that as soon as he put his hands on the string, the sound engineer's equipment started to pick up high frequency sound waves. How can a piece of string with a small piece of wood on the end give off high frequency sound waves? Try this at home for yourselves. I am sure that the kind of equipment to pick up high frequency sound waves is much cheaper now than it was in the 1960s. Your teenager may even have something that can do this, and he or she will have the time to experiment even if you don't. You can make this device in minutes. All you need is a block of wood cut to a size of about one inch by half an inch, or one third of an inch. Draw across the two diagonals to find the center, and then drill a small hole with a wood drill through the center. Then thread a piece of string fifty inches long through the piece of wood, and wrap the other end around a ballpoint pen. Roll the string up until it is approximately 31.5 inches long, put a steel table knife either on the floor or on a table, and then move the string very slowly either side of the 31.5 inch point, and when you get exactly the right length the weight will start to move. This is easier to see if you have someone hold the piece of wood still, and then the string will vibrate when you have the right length (you can also hold the piece of wood yourself if your arms are long enough). My guess is that somewhere between 10% and 50% of you will be able to do this, and if you try it and succeed then it will open your eyes to another world. I have no idea how that works. I just know that it does, and that it is easily duplicated.

I had a Computer Science teacher once from Eastern Europe who was able to make a steel bus stop vibrate so much that it almost pulled out of the ground, and he did it just by using a small tuning fork. I wish I knew how he did this, unfortunately he didn't tell us, but what he did say was that when he was fifteen, he would almost cause car crashes because drivers would drive by and see a fifteen year old boy standing quietly next to a steel bus stop that was waving backwards and forwards like a tree in a high wind. He was one of the brightest men I ever met. He taught us computer science at university, and I wish I could have sat down with him and talked more about some of the things he could do.

To give you another example of energy fields, I was once with two friends in Glastonbury in England. Glastonbury is one of the supposed possible sites for the court of King Arthur, and it is an interesting place to visit. It is also somewhat of a New Age center too. My friends and I were walking near Glastonbury Tor, which is a small hill about 500 feet high. A foreign woman with a small group around her asked if we could help with something they were doing. We were fine with that, and she told us all to stand in a circle. She told us to cross our arms across our chests, and link hands with the person next to us so I linked my right hand to the hand of the person on my left, and my left hand to the hand of the person on my right. She taught us a four line chorus, and said that she would do the rest of the chant, and all we had to do was join in the chorus. She stood in the middle of the circle, and started to chant while the group circled around her. This lasted maybe five to ten minutes with the chant getting louder and faster. At the end she threw her arms up in the air, and we had all been instructed to do the same. She had told us to make sure our hands remained linked, and the circle wasn't broken. I threw my arms in the air, keeping hold of the hands of the person either side of me, and everyone else did the same. At the moment we threw our hands up, all chanting and all movement stopped and we were rooted to the spot, and what happened next was fascinating. I felt a wave of energy come up from the ground through my feet, moving up through my body, and then out through the top of my head. Let's say this again because there is no way science can explain this - I felt a wave of energy come up from the ground through my feet, moving up through my body, and then out through the top of my head.

This was not a slight feeling or something I may, or may not, have felt. It was a distinctive wave of force. Three other people felt it too, but the rest of the group did not. I was stunned, and said so, and that was when I found out that only a few of us had felt it. We were not told to expect this, and I had no idea it was going to happen. I had no ill effects from it, and when I asked the foreign woman about it she casually said that some people felt something, and others did not. Then she thanked us for participating, and we went on our way. The big question is, what the heck happened, what was the wave of force, and how was it generated? How can people dance in a circle and chant, and then something like that happens? Five years of physics at school, tells me that some kind of force was generated, but the question is what? It was not electrical or static in any way because there were none of the effects you get if you hold onto a Van de Graaf generator, but there was no question something happened. If anyone knows what this is or how it was generated, then I would love to hear from you. Once again, my email address is at the back of the book.

I used these examples just to illustrate that there are things in this world which just cannot be explained by Western science. If you start looking then things like this are all over the place. I have a scientific mind, and I am fascinated by some of the anomalies in our world. What I am trying to say by this is that yoga and Tai Chi may well be more than just exercises. I have done a fair amount of yoga, and a few years ago practiced it every day for a year and a half. I am just starting to read up on Tai Chi and I intend to experiment with it, and one of the interesting things with that is that the books tells you to imagine energy moving through your body as you do the exercise, and the books I have read state that you will only get the true benefits if you do that.

Let me tell you how I got onto this path of open-mindedness about science, although it may well be that I just had it in me, to be that way. When I was a teenager I used to watch a science program on the BBC called "Tomorrow's World". It was a great program, and many people watched it. There was a presenter called Michael Rodd, and one day the show opened with him standing by a river in the Chicago area. I have a really good visual memory, and I can still see Michael Rodd standing there in my mind's eye. It was sunny, and he stood on grass and between him and the river were a series of metal coat hangers, straightened out and standing upright in the sun. Bear in mind this was a science program, and I was expecting something scientific. Michael Rodd then went on to explain that the sun shining on the metal rods was casting shadows on the ground. He pulled the metal coat hangers out of the ground, and then explained that even though the metal rods had been removed, their shadows would leave something in the ground that would decay like a radioactive half life, and that a dowser would be able to pick this up with a dowsing rod. He said it would fade in about three days, and would get fainter every day. To say that I was stunned was an understatement. I had not expected to see anything like that. I decided then and there that I would investigate, and read about the kind of things like this, that science did not normally accept, and that is the approach I have taken for the whole of my life. There is a lot of false information out there, and a lot of garbage, but there is also stuff that cannot possibly be explained by Western science, and we should look out for that and question it. Many scientists have their salaries paid for by groups other than the university they work at, and often they do not want to rock the boat, but an ordinary person like you or I can easily question things like that.

I once saw a video that was made near a crop circle in England. The people who made the video were just talking, and filming it for their records, but while they were talking they noticed a bright light circling above the crop circle. They were wondering what this was, and asking if anyone saw it (it was plainly visible on the film) when a British military helicopter came roaring over the horizon. It headed straight for the circle of light, but it was obvious that the men in the helicopter were being guided by radio, and didn't actually know where the circle of light was. They went straight past it, and on the film the circle moved out of the way to avoid the helicopter, and they went off in the wrong direction. A few seconds later they made a sharp turn and came roaring back, but it was obvious again that the men in the helicopter were being guided towards the light by someone who had it on radar, rather than homing in on it themselves. Shortly after that the light just vanished, but the point is that it must have given off some kind of electro-magnetic radiation that the military was able to detect, and all this was captured on film. Had the British military helicopter not appeared and chased after the light, then all that would have been there would have been a light dancing around on a film, which in theory anybody could have added to the negatives if they were so inclined, but the actions of the military helicopter gave the whole video an entirely different dimension.

Let's take a look at yoga first. There are many different kinds of yoga. The type I did was Baron Baptiste Power Vinyasa Yoga. I had looked at several different types of yoga and I have a lot of books on yoga, and Baron Baptiste's book was the one that I preferred. Baptiste is the son of two early yoga practitioners from California, which means he has been around yoga for the whole of his life. I have several of his DVDs, and at the start of one of them Baron moves in and out of different positions making them seem effortless. Baptiste's yoga will give you a really good workout. You can do it at home, or you can do it at a class. You can find yoga teachers all over the United States, and I know there is a program that teaches Baptiste's Power Vinyasa Yoga. There is at least one in Jacksonville near where I live, and they are all over the United States.

Baptiste's Power Vinyasa Yoga falls into what is often described as "hot yoga", in that it is done in a warm room. We live in Florida, and when I did it in the summer I would often open the double doors onto the patio from our bedroom, and let the Florida heat in while I worked out. One of the great things about Baptiste's book is that you can read the book, and then just go ahead and do it. There are some difficult poses, but one thing Baron does is give you modified poses, which you can do instead of the main pose that will get you partway there. There is absolutely no point in straining yourself, or injuring yourself just to get a pose that is the same way as someone from India could do it. Baptiste's poses are easier to do than some of the ones in some other yoga books, and at the end of the day you will get a lot of benefits. Once again, I am going to say buy Baron Baptiste's book, just the same as I told you to buy Arnold's book, or Tosca Reno's book. If you buy a book written by someone who has been doing his particular sport or type of yoga for a long time, and follow it then you are far less likely to injure yourself than if you follow a different path. It is always important to take things a little slower, and not get injured than it is to plunge in too quickly, and spend the next two weeks flat on your back in bed. There is some great advice in Baron Baptiste's book, and it is well worth buying this one. Once again, it is called "Journey Into Power : How to Sculpt Your Ideal Body, Free your True Self and Transform your Life with Baptiste Power Vinyasa Yoga".

One thing that is important with yoga, or with any other exercise, is the following. There is one yoga person out there who tells you to drop all other exercises including running, and weight lifting, and anything else you do, and only do his type of yoga. I have to advise against this. If you see a statement like this whether it is about exercise, or food, or something else, I don't think you should follow it. I would never turn round and say to anyone to follow what is in this book, and drop everything else you are doing. With any book or any system what you should do is read the book, and incorporate it into what you already have. I am not going to name anyone who states in their books to drop all other exercises, but it is something to look out for and to guard against. The same goes for diets. If anyone tells you to throw all the food out in your pantry, buy their food, and eat only what they tell you to eat in their book then watch out for your health because you may be about to lose it.

Tai Chi and Qigong

Nissan was the first Japanese car company to set up shop in Britain. One of the big things that journalists wrote about was the fact that the workers at the Nissan plants in Japan did exercises every morning before they started work, usually in the fresh air outside the factory. The British papers did not think that British workers should be subjected to this. I was young at the time this happened, but I thought that they had missed a golden opportunity. It would be interesting if they had done this, and then found that workers at the Nissan plant suffered fewer heart attacks, and were healthier than workers at other British car plants. Since it was stopped we don't know whether this would have happened, but I think if they had done that they could have made a major change to British culture. Even if they had just said that the exercises would be voluntary, and said that anybody who wanted could do them, they would have probably found that many people would have drifted into them albeit with a lot of jokes.

Life for an old person is very different in Japan, than it is the United States and Britain. A Japanese person is usually flexible, and able to walk right through old age, and only becomes infirm a year or two before he or she dies. In the West people can often be infirm for twenty years before they die, and to be quite honest there is no need for that. I was talking to a physical therapist yesterday and he told me that synovial fluid, which is the fluid that lubricates the joints, is released when the joints are moved. So if you exercise a lot your joints become used to releasing a lot of lubricant, whereas if you sit around a lot and spend your days watching television then less lubricant is released into your joints, and they are subject to more wear. We are often told that older people have painful joints because they have overused them in their lifetimes, but what if it is the other way round? What if their joints are painful because they have underused them, and the joints did not release as much synovial fluid to lubricate themselves?

There are many things that can damage joints such as using them in an unnatural way, and you have to think about that too. I once got onto an elliptical machine when they first came out, but I only used it for a few minutes because I felt that my back was moving in an unnatural way. If you do that you may wear out a joint over time. I try and stick to movements that our ancestors would have done ten thousand years ago. Like I said before, walking is a normal movement, but swinging your arms in an exaggerated manner to try and burn more energy is not a natural movement, so think about it before you do it. Would it not be better to just walk for ten minutes longer, and burn more energy that way than to do the exaggerated arm movements and damage something?

Very little is known about Tai Chi in the West. If I had known that Tai Chi was originally developed from exercises used to strengthen the body for martial arts, I would have taken a much greater interest in it at an earlier date. Somehow in the West it is assumed that Tai Chi is an exercise purely for old Asian people, which is a very naïve viewpoint. I am sure I will get a lot of letters now from people who tell me that Tai Chi is nothing like that. However, this is the viewpoint I held for many years, and I got that viewpoint from what is in the Western media. There is a Tai Chi studio literally two miles from our house, and my wife and I have often passed that studio and thought about going in, but we have not done this and the reason may have been a lack of understanding about what Tai Chi actually is.

The only reason I started to look into Tai Chi is that there is a library at the halfway point on one of my five mile walks, and this summer it was so hot in Jacksonville that I started going into the library to cool off for five or ten minutes before going back out.

One day I picked up a book on Tai Chi by an Asian Australian called Gary Khor, and there was a wealth of wisdom in that book. One of the things he said was that as you get older the blood flow to your joints diminishes, and the exercises for Tai Chi help to increase blood flow to the joints. Now this is important, why are we not told in the West that the blood flow to your joints diminishes as you get older? If you know about something then you can do something about it. One of the reasons I walk so much is that I want to make sure that when I am old, I will have good blood circulation in my legs, and if I walk a lot then that is much more likely to happen than if I watch television for three hours every night.

If you do happen to be a person who watches television for three hours every night then every bit of exercise you do from now on can improve your circulation. It is never too late. Believe it or not there are quite a few ninety year olds doing yoga, and they probably put a lot of fifty year olds to shame. My mother used to do a lot of "keep fit", which was basically a set of exercises they used to do in Britain when I was young. She kept that up, and one day when we went to visit her when she was 80 years old, she stood up and demonstrated that she could still touch her toes. My mother was definitely an 18 year old trapped in an 80 year old body.

Actually, there is something we should think about here. It often seems to me that mammals have been short changed when it comes to aging. Captain James Cook presented the King of Tonga with a giant tortoise on his voyage in 1777, and that tortoise lived until 1965 and was estimated to be 188 years old when it died. How can a tortoise live to be 188 years old when a mouse lasts just three years? There is an inconsistency here somewhere that cannot be explained by the standard explanation that people and animals age because their bodies slowly decay. Somewhere in the body there must be a clock, and if that clock exists then there is a possibility that it can be stopped or even reset.

There is a class of animals called "Monotremes" from Australia. Monotremes have hair and give their young milk, and have quite a lot of mammal characteristics, but they also lay eggs. The spiny anteater is a monotreme, and so is the duck billed platypus. The spiny anteater (Short-Beaked Echidna) is 12 inches to 18 inches long, and can live to be 50 years old. It lays one egg a year, and can wait between two to six years before reproducing again. Contrast this with a mammal of the same size that pushes out as many young as possible, and lives less than five years. The duck billed platypus does not live as long as the spiny anteater, and has only lived to be 17 years old in zoos. An interesting fact is that the platypus locates its prey by detecting electrical fields generated by muscle contractions in the animal they are stalking. This is called electroreception.

It seems to me that the way mammals rose to dominate the Earth was to develop short life spans, and breed very fast. Compared to some reptiles we are gone in an instant. There is a very rare disease called "Progeria", which affects one person in eight million (numbers vary on this from one person in four million, to one person in 44 million). With this disease, children begin to show signs of aging by the time they reach their first birthdays. They do not age in exactly the same way that normal people age, in that some of the signs of aging are missing, but what does happen is that their bodies age much faster than the bodies of normal people. It is possible that when we understand exactly how progeria works we may understand how normal aging works, and perhaps at that point we will be able to switch it off. It is quite possible in my opinion that aging is held off until a certain age, and then just ticks off according to a clock somewhere in the body. It seems to me that the body's repair mechanisms are just slowly shut down until something important breaks and we die.

I said all this because I don't think we have any real understanding of the process of aging. Certain things seem to tick off according to a prearranged clock. If I ever say this to anyone they will immediately tell me that people age at different rates, and that much is definitely true. Live a hard life and abuse your body, and you will look a lot older at fifty, than someone who has led a clean life. We can turn this around though too. If you lead a cleaner life, then maybe your body's repair mechanisms can more easily cope with repairing some of the damage that can be done to the body as we get older. If you are twenty, then your body can pretty much repair itself whatever you do to it, whereas if you are seventy and you do the some of the things that twenty year old

Americans routinely do to their bodies, then you may not wake up the next morning.

I have heard from quite a few sources that practicing yoga or Tai Chi can hold off aging to some extent. I was once asked by an English colleague who did yoga how old I thought she was. I am not keen on doing this because if you get it wrong then you will not be a popular person. I thought she was mid forties, but I knocked a few years off anyway just to be on the safe side, and she told me she was more than ten years older than I had guessed which surprised me. She attributed that to a practice of yoga. There is a system called "The Five Tibetans" that seems to be based on yoga positions, and it claims to do something similar. I tried that at one time and my wife told me I looked younger the same night I started doing it, which was interesting because I hadn't told her I was doing it, and to be honest such a claim sounded a bit farfetched to me. It is well worth checking this out, and the book I used is "The Five Tibetans" by Christopher Kilham. This is a concise, easy to read book, and I can definitely recommend it. As always follow the instructions carefully to avoid injury. If you have plenty of funds then it is well worth buying "The Ancient Secret of the Fountain of Youth" by Peter Kelder, which gives a little more detail although I have to say I prefer the book by Christopher Kilham. The books by Peter Kelder are apparently incredibly popular in Germany, and sell very well over there.

The Five Tibetans will probably take you ten to fifteen minutes, and I found them to have good effects. Once again I see something here when I am writing about it, and think that I need to get back to it. I have done the Five Tibetans on and off many times over the years. The reason I keep saying I must get back to a certain type of exercise is that I have done so many different exercises over the years that I could fill a whole week every week if I did everything. I remember reading about a man when I was a teenager. This man was seventy years old, and most men died before that age when I was a teenager. He attributed his health and longevity to the fact that he walked to the end of his garden every morning, jumped in the river, and swam quite a long way up river before turning, and swimming back down river. He did this every day of the year except on Christmas Day, and if you have never been to England then anyone who is prepared to jump into an

English river in the middle of winter wearing just swimming trunks has to be tough. Again, this is a case of use it or lose it. If you tried jumping in a river, and doing that at age seventy, the result may well be a trip to the hospital in an ambulance, but if you do it from when you are relatively young it is amazing what the body can do.

The book I found in my local library by Gary Khor about Tai Chi was very interesting, and also very informative. I already mentioned the point about blood flow to the joints, but one of the other things Khor mentioned, was that the blood circulation in the body is controlled by three areas, the heart, the lungs, and the muscles in the body. He then went on to say that if your muscles are developed, and not slack, then they will push the blood through the body thus taking some of the pressure off the heart. The first thing I think of when I hear that is why aren't we told that in the West? The instant I read that I could immediately see the benefits of having your muscles in good shape. Most books on Tai Chi tell you that you should see some benefits within a month of starting to do the exercises. The two main books I have on Tai Chi are "Tai Chi for Stress Control and Relaxation" by Gary Khor, and "Chinese Fitness: A Mind/Body Approach – Qigong for Healthy and Joyful Living" by Qingshan Liu. Qingshan Liu is a qigong teacher who lives in Munich, Germany. I actually bought his book several years ago in the Chinese store at Disney in Orlando, Florida. I read it at the time, but I was in a job that paid a lot of money but left me with very little energy outside work, and it is only recently that I picked it up and looked at it again. The exercises in this book are similar in some ways, to the ones in Gary Khor's book, and I will probably do both sets before settling on one or the other.

I cannot speak from experience about Tai Chi or Qigong yet because I have not really gotten into them, apart from working through some of Gary Khor's book, and working through some of the moves on a Tai Chi DVD called "T'ai Chi Beginning Practice by David Dorian Ross who is American. This is a DVD that you can watch just for relaxation. It is a Gaiam DVD. One thing I have found about Gaiam DVDs is that you have to be careful not to overdo things if you do the exercises. I have a few Rodney Yee yoga DVDs by them, and when I watched them, I could see that it was way above my level. The Tai Chi DVD seemed simpler, but it did cause me to have a minor injury in one of the movements where you cross your arms across your body. This was nothing major and cleared up after a couple of days. My first boss when I came to America once made the comment that most bad injuries usually clear to a large extent after 48 hours. I had never heard this before, but I took note, and he was exactly right, you can be in pretty bad shape with an injury, but if you can wait 48 hours then often a lot of the pain is gone.

If you are older, or infirm, and want to exercise then there is a book called "Tai Chi in a Chair" by Cynthia Quarta that may well be worth buying. Here is the Amazon link to the book:

http://www.amazon.com/dp/193141260X/

One thing I am going to do to a certain extent with this book is make it an interactive book. Like I said earlier, I have not really tried Tai Chi, or Qigong to the extent I can comment on it properly. If anyone out there has a lot of experience with Tai Chi or Qigong, and feels they have they have something to add here, then please write to me at the email address at the back of the book, and if I think it is something would be useful to enter then I will add it, maybe as an appendix. I am a great believer that nobody should have to reinvent the wheel. We, as a race, spend far too much time duplicating things that other people have already done. One of the reasons we are here, and not some other species of human, is that our ancestors when they were nomads, were willing to share any new discovery and often to share food too. The first Neanderthal skeleton was discovered by a German scientist, and "thal" means "valley" in German. Thus, Neanderthal Man means Neander Valley Man in German. This is interesting because in the ice age all the places with the mildest climates (in a Europe that looked a lot like the North Pole) were the valleys, and Neanderthal Men had all the valleys, and Cro-Magnon Men were stuck with the ridges, and the hills. So at the start of the ice age, Neanderthal Men had the best places to live, which suggests they were dominant, but by the end of the ice age they were gone from Europe, and our ancestors were still there. The last Neanderthal found in Europe was a young girl, who was living with a family of Cro-Magnons, when they all died in a cave on the Iberian

Peninsula (Spain). Everyone in the world who is not pure African has 1% to 4% of Neanderthal genes, and it is likely that the ancestors of modern humans met Neanderthals just after they left Africa, and intermingled with them. We are used to thinking of ourselves as the smartest or dominant human, but Cro-Magnon Men had bigger brains than we do, and it is possible that some Neanderthal Men did too, as their cranial capacity was at least as big as ours, and may have been larger. Remember that it is not always the smartest human that survives, it is the one with the biggest club, and the one who is prepared to use that club.

The Neanderthals who lived in Europe had a dormant gene switched on (at least it is dormant in us), which promoted excessive bone growth, which is one of the reasons they looked a lot different than we do. It is possible that this was a reaction due to the ice age. The southern Neanderthal, which lived in the Middle East around Israel, and probably other areas, looked more like modern humans than the European Neanderthal because it did not have the gene turned on that promoted excessive bone growth.

I have heard it said by quite a few people, that Neanderthal Men could not speak, but this is plainly ridiculous. Genetic analysis indicates that they had exactly the same version of the FOXP2 gene that we do, which is the gene that is associated with speech. Having a descended hyoid bone also allows us to speak, and although I don't know whether Neanderthal men had descended hyoid bones, I would assume that they did. The hyoid bone is the only bone in the human body that is not connected to any other bone, and if a pathologist finds a broken hyoid bone on a dead body, then it is almost certain that person was strangled as that is just about the only way to break the hyoid bone. The FOXP2 gene is on Chromosome 7 in a human.

I will talk more about human DNA in a later chapter, as that may be one of the reasons we are so prone to diabetes. There is less genetic variation in the entire human race than in just one group of chimpanzees, so at sometime in the distant past there were only a very few of us. Genetics indicates that there were definitely less than 5,000 of us, and there may have been considerably less than that. More about that in a later chapter.

Glucose Transporters and Human DNA

In this chapter I want to talk about glucose transporters and human DNA, and I will look at glucose transporters first. What I'm primarily interested in here is an increase in glucose transport into muscles because the more glucose your muscles can pull in, the less glucose there will be in your blood. I want to look at a study conducted at the Washington University School of Medicine in St. Louis, Missouri back in 2006. However, first let's take a quick look at glucose transporters. I am not going to get too technical here so don't worry if one paragraph sounds that way, the rest will be easy to read.

Glucose transporters are a group of membrane proteins that facilitate the transport of glucose over a cell membrane. There are three classes of glucose transporters with the main ones falling into Class I. Glucose transporters GLUT 1, GLUT 2, GLUT 3 and GLUT 4 all fall into Class I. If you want to look up the gene card for these glucose transporters then the code for GLUT 1 is SLC2A1 and the gene card for GLUT 2 is SLC2A2, and so on. I usually look them up at the Weizmann Institute of Science, which provides a database that can be accessed by the public. The SLC2 part of the gene card stands for "solute carrier family 2". I will try not to make this too technical, although if anyone is interested in getting really technical then please email me at the email address at the back of the book, and I will provide you the web links I used to write this part of the book.

Okay, that should be the main technical sounding part over. Thirteen glucose transporters have been identified so far, and all this has been relatively recent since the late 1980s. I am going to stick with the first class of glucose transporters for now. What is important here is that we are told that insulin resistance is one of the primary causes of type 2 diabetes. That is a fair enough comment, but there are two pathways for glucose transport into muscles. The first pathway is triggered by insulin, and the second pathway is triggered either by muscle contractions, or by hypoxia (shortage of oxygen). The second pathway is one we can work with, and here is how we do that.

Muscle contractions induce an increase in glucose transport, and in this case GLUT 4 is the glucose transporter that transports glucose into the muscles. The acute effect of muscle contractions on glucose transport is completely independent of insulin, and it reverses rapidly after exercise stops. Now here is the interesting part, once exercise stops the muscles are left much more sensitive to insulin. Scientists do not yet know why this occurs, but it does it occur, and it can be measured. It appears that this is caused by translocation of more GLUT 4 to the surfaces of the cells.

One thing I just cannot talk about too much here is that this is a tipping point. Effectively what is happening here is that the muscle cells are now much more sensitive to insulin. This won't last, and they will return to normal in the near future, but what you have is a situation where the muscle is eager to pull sugar out of your bloodstream, and you are in a situation where you are very eager to have sugar pulled out of your bloodstream so for you, and for your muscles, this is a win win situation.

Now I said earlier that scientists don't know why this happens, but let's take a step back, and apply a little common sense. Say it is 25,000 years ago, and you are a seventeen year old male armed with a wooden spear with a stone point. Two other hunters flank you, but you're the fastest. Ahead of you is a deer. The three of you are wearing it down. It is already injured, but you are approaching wolf territory, and if you don't catch it then all the effort you have put in will be gone, and you will have just provided breakfast for the wolves. The three of you could follow the deer into wolf territory, but you know full well that if you do that then you will be providing the wolves not only with breakfast, but also with lunch, and all that will be left of you will be your stone spear. You have been running for half an hour at a steady trot, and so has the deer. Your muscles have used up all their stored sugar, and are demanding sugar from your bloodstream. Do you think at that point your muscles will be extra sensitive to insulin so that they can pull sugar from your blood stream? You can bet they will, and you can also bet that there are GLUT 4 transporters working like crazy to pull sugar out of your bloodstream. The deer puts on a burst of speed. You look at the two other hunters, and you know that they are almost spent. As the fastest it is up to you to make the kill. You put on one last desperate burst of speed and take the deer down. Ahead of you on the ridge line stands a single solitary wolf. He hasn't seen you yet so you pull the deer swiftly behind a tree and go in behind it. Either side of you the other two hunters duck into cover. You look at the other two and exchange a glance, and a quick smile. Victory is yours. You will eat tonight.

Flash forward 25,000 years. You are seventeen years old. There are cases of beer on the table in the kitchen, and your father and his friends are in the family room watching the game. You and your friends duck into the kitchen. They flank you on either side, but you are the fastest. You grab one case of beer, and the three of you duck into the garage. You have made it without being caught. Victory is yours. The sound of three cans popping comes all at once. You pull back your head, and down half of the first can. The beer tastes good as it goes down.

Given the two lives, I'd rather be the seventeen year old who lived 25,000 years ago, but maybe I'm a little different. He is probably far more alive than his descendant will ever be. You see from the first example though how we're wired to pull sugar out of our bloodstreams. The study conducted at the Washington University School of Medicine in St. Louis, Missouri back in 2006, was really looking at whether a jolt of insulin would make the muscles more sensitive to insulin later on, but the results of the study indicated that any of the three factors, muscle contractions, hypoxia, or insulin would bring about increased sensitivity to insulin for a short period in the muscles. We are approaching it from a completely different direction than the researchers were because they were looking at it from the point of view of extra insulin (at least that was my impression on reading the study). We are looking at things from the point of view of lowering the sugar in our bloodstreams. This is interesting because when I first started attacking type 2 diabetes, what I did was to begin exercising within fifteen minutes of finishing a meal. I did this because I was aiming to reduce the amount of insulin in my bloodstream. This is different than aiming to reduce the amount of sugar in your blood because if you did that, then it wouldn't matter when you started exercising. If you aim to reduce the amount of insulin, then starting exercise as quickly as possible does two things. Firstly it starts to reduce the amount of sugar in your blood, which, in theory, should mean less insulin is pumped out. This may not happen the first time, but your body is not stupid, it will learn quickly that you are going to exercise after every meal or at least after the ones you take at home, and it will act accordingly.

Like I said earlier, I don't want to get too technical and go into massive detail about this study because believe I will switch at least half the readers off if I do that. I can provide you with the web link to download the report. Let's look at the glucose transporters in Class I now. Glucose transporter 1 (GLUT 1) is responsible for pulling small amounts of glucose into cells in the body to keep them ticking over (if that is the right word). GLUT 1 is also the channel for vitamin C to enter the bodies of mammals that cannot make it for themselves. Your dog or cat cannot get scurvy because they make vitamin C in their bodies. Years ago when I was young, I used to wonder how meat eating animals such as dogs and cats got vitamin C into their bodies, and then one day I read that they made it. Presumably we don't make it because most primates are surrounded by tons of vitamin C, but that does make it difficult for any primate that leaves the trees, and stops eating fruit and other foods that contain vitamin C. GLUT 1 is also used by the Human T-lymphotropic virus (HTLV) to gain entry into cells in the body. HTLV-I is a retrovirus, and is made up of two copies of an RNA virus, whose genome is copied into a double stranded DNA form that integrates into the host cell genome. If HTLV-I gets that far into your body then you are in serious trouble, and some people who get this virus get cancer.

If you remember in the introduction I stated that the next super weapon will probably be an RNA virus. I am no top flight geneticist, but half an hour's research on Wikipedia found me an RNA virus that can be pulled into the body by a glucose transporter, GLUT 1, that goes to pretty much every cell in the body. I am sure there are many governments around the world that could take HTLV-1, analyze its genome if it hasn't already been published, and then either tweak it or produce their own RNA virus using the properties that allow it to be transported by GLUT 1. The big advantage of an RNA virus is that you don't have to give it life, if you make your own DNA virus then you have to kick a number of processes off together to give it life, whereas with an RNA virus you just make the virus, and then put it into a target cell and off it goes. In 2010 the Chinese company BGI (formerly

Beijing Genomics Institute) acquired 128 new Illumina HiSeq 2000 genome sequencers. BGI is based in Shenzhen, China and it installed 100 of the gene sequencing machines in a building in Hong Kong to work with Western companies. Like I said earlier, this one building in Hong Kong has more gene sequencing capability than exists in the whole of the United States, or at least it did in 2010. Hopefully this has now been rectified, but any American university that wants one of these machines should have one in my opinion. If we don't do that, we risk falling behind. GLUT 1 is encoded by the SLC2A1 gene, which is located on chromosome 1 on a human.

Let's look at glucose transporter 2 (GLUT 2) now. GLUT 2 is what is known as a bi-directional transporter. It allows glucose to flow in two directions. It is the main glucose transporter that allows glucose to be moved between the bloodstream and the liver, and it also works in the beta cells in the pancreas, and in the renal tubular cells (kidneys). GLUT 2 also carries glucosamine, which helps the joints. GLUT 2 is encoded by the SLC2A2 gene, which is located on chromosome 3 on a human.

Glucose transporter 3 (GLUT 3) is the main glucose transporter for the neurons in the brain. GLUT 3 has a greater glucose carrying capacity than any of the other three glucose transporters in Class I, which it would have to have because if your brain runs out of sugar, you are done. Some of the poisons mankind uses actually work by blocking the uptake of sugar into cells, and the creature targeted dies, in many cases, surrounded by an abundance of food. GLUT 3 is encoded by the SLC2A3 gene, which is located on chromosome 12 on a human.

Glucose transporter 4 (GLUT 4) is the insulin regulated glucose transporter involved in glucose transport into fat tissue (adipose tissue), and also into striated muscles (skeletal muscles and heart muscles). I have talked a lot about GLUT 4 in other parts of this book so I won't repeat it again here. GLUT 4 is encoded by the SLC2A4 gene, which is located on chromosome 17 on a human.

Much more is known about the Class I glucose transporters than Class II and III. Glucose transporter 5 (GLUT 5) is the first transporter in Class II, and it is a fructose transporter. GLUT 5 exists in muscles, but in a study published at the US National

Library of Medicine there is a comment that while muscle inactivity caused a significant reduction in muscle GLUT 4 expression, it had no detectable effects on GLUT 5. What this means for our purposes, in plain English, is that working your muscles will rev up glucose transporter 4 to pull sugar out of your bloodstream and into your muscles, whereas glucose transporter 5 does not appear to get the same push from muscle activity. The main conclusion of this report indicated that further research was needed, in that the muscles have a fructose transporter present (GLUT 5) that can be used to transport fructose into muscle cells, but muscle activity does not stimulate this in the same way it stimulates GLUT 4 to pull in more glucose. Thus it would almost seem that GLUT 5 is present in muscles just in case only fructose is available, and not glucose (my words not the researchers). Glucose is one of the main products of photosynthesis. Glucose and fructose have exactly the same chemical formula ($C_6H_{12}O_6$) but they have different structures. Scientists do not understand why glucose is used in organisms instead of fructose or another monosaccharide. GLUT 5 is encoded by the SLC2A5 gene, which is located on chromosome 1 on a human.

That is pretty much what I have on glucose transporters. Research is still ongoing, and only Class 1 has been extensively researched. It has recently been discovered that glucose transporter 9 (GLUT 9) transports uric acid in the kidneys. GLUT 9 is encoded by the SLC2A9 gene, which is located on chromosome 4 on a human. Genetic variants of the SLC2A9 gene have been linked to increased risk of hyperuricemia (high level of uric acid in the blood) and gout.

Human DNA

I have said before that the entire human race is descended from a very small root population. Something happened in the last 100,000 years, where there were there were only a few people left in the human population. It is actually possible that we are descended from just two people according to a leading geneticist, and it is extremely likely that we are descended from less than 5,000 people. Let's look at an example from the squirrel population. In the 1870s, one hundred American eastern gray squirrels were introduced into the UK. Their descendants now number around two million squirrels, and because they store fat more easily and are fitter than the UK native red squirrel, they have replaced the red squirrel in much of the UK. A genetic analysis of the British gray squirrel would look like the human gene analysis, in that it would show that they are descended from a small root population. Somehow our ancestors either became separated from the rest of their group, and prospered, and changed or most of humanity was wiped out, and they were all that were left. The result is us.

Genetic analysis using mitochondrial DNA can tell us a lot. Sometime in the past, Melanesians from Papua New Guinea colonized the island of Fiji. We know that the boats that took Melanesians to Fiji contained mostly women from the lowlands of Papua New Guinea, but genetic analysis shows that 18% of the population of Fiji is descended from women from the highlands of Papua New Guinea. I mentioned earlier in this book that I have a book called "Pacific: The boundless Ocean" by French author Alain Chenevière, which is basically about Polynesia. Chenevière covers multiple islands in the book peopled by Melanesians, and Polynesians, and one thing that is obvious is that the people of the islands are a real mix. There are people on some islands who look as though they could have come straight from Asia, and other people who look pure Melanesian, as though they are descended from Papua New Guineans. Before genetic analysis existed, languages were used to plot Polynesian migration routes. American author Paul Theroux traveled through the Pacific, and he commented that many of the islanders are now scared of going on the water and get seasick easily, which is interesting considering that their ancestors were such incredible sailors.

One of the interesting things that has been discovered in just the last five years, is that up to 6% of the DNA of Melanesians and Australian aborigines comes from a hitherto unknown species of human, meaning that not only do people outside Africa have 1% to 4% of Neanderthal genes in them, but there is also a third human ancestor to consider. In 2008 scientists from the Institute of Archaeology and Ethnology of Novosibirsk, uncovered a finger from a juvenile female of a new species of human that has since been named Denisovan Man, or Denisovan Woman, after the Denisova cave in the Altai Mountains in Siberia where the finger was discovered. The find has been dated to 41,000 years ago.

The nearest city to the Denisova cave is Barnaul, which is 150 miles (241 kilometers) south of Novosibirsk. Novosibirsk is a Russian city in Siberia, and is a major stop on the Trans-Siberian Railroad. In the days of the Russian Empire, the Russians used to build the Russian settlement next to the old settlement that was already there, and you can find that in all the old Khanates which the Russians took down in the eighteenth and nineteenth centuries. During one of their great expansions, the Russian army conquered an area the size of Europe in just ten years, which was an incredible achievement. To a certain extent Russian frontier towns were a lot like the Wild West in America, and they must have been interesting places to visit. There is a really interesting book by Anton Chekhov called "A Journey to the End of the Russian Empire", where Chekhov journeyed to Sakhalin Island, which is on Russia's far eastern seaboard. The Trans-Siberian had not been built at the time, and it was quite a tough trip for Chekhov, and it makes for fascinating reading.

It is not just in ancient times that small populations became isolated. I have a book called "Tibet: The Secret Continent" by Frenchman Michel Peissel. On page 64 of the book is a section called "The Faces of Tibet". On that page is an inhabitant of Tibet who would not look out of place in Britain, in fact, he could very easily pass for an Englishman, and could definitely pass for a North European. Every other face on the page is an Asian face. The man with the European face is a Minaro. The Minaro are now confined to six valleys, which dead end at one end and are easily defended at the other end, which is why they are still there. If there were no Europeans, and the ancestors of Europeans had been wiped out by another race, then the Minaro could quite easily be the only remnants of an archaic race of humans. Because in the past mankind has moved long distances in relatively short time frames, it is easy to find examples like that. In many places in Asia and Indonesia there are hill tribes who are of a different race than the Asians that now surround them. Indonesia has now sent Indonesian colonists to Irian Jaya, which is the Indonesian half of the island of New Guinea. If human civilization were to collapse tomorrow, then in 10,000 years the descendants of those Indonesian settlers may well make up the major part of the population of New Guinea, with the Melanesians having retreated to the high areas that are hard to get to.

One point I should make about the Minaro, which I mentioned above, is that they are closely related to the Iranian race. However, many Westerners don't realize how closely the Iranians are related to North West Europeans. In the Iranian language, the word "Iran" means "Land (or place) of the Aryans". One thing you may not know is that the closest modern language to ancient Sanskrit is not actually modern Hindi as you might expect, in fact, modern Lithuanian is actually closer to Sanskrit than modern Hindi is. The Lithuanians were the last nation to be Christianized in Europe, and their ancient Gods correspond closely with the ancient Gods of the Iranians, and the Gods of the Hindus in India. One of the other interesting things I have read is that there is speculation that Sanskrit was an invented language because it is so regular. I am not qualified to comment on that, but we have Esperanto, which was a language made up in the twentieth century with the intention that everyone in the world should be taught Esperanto, so that people would only have to learn one language. It was a good idea that never caught on. The American Science Fiction author Harry Harrison is fluent in Esperanto, and often uses Esperanto phrases in his books. Of course, if Sanskrit really is a made up language, then that means there was an advanced civilization in the fairly recent past, which we now have absolutely no knowledge of.

I find it hard to believe that a species that is descended from primates can have any kind of problem with blood sugar. Our primate ancestors must have eaten huge quantities of fruit. It is likely that our limited genome is the problem. If we are descended from a very small root population, and one of those ancestors had a problem with blood sugar, then that problem is in all of us. There are all kinds of problems that pop up all over the world from inbreeding, but I would be willing to bet that the chances of similar problems popping up in chimpanzee populations are much smaller because of their wide genetic variation. I remember when I was young they used to show multiple programs on television about World War II, and it always struck me when they covered the Japanese army, how many young Japanese men wore glasses compared with the British population, where it is unusual to see a young man in his twenties with glasses. Somewhere in the ancestry of the Japanese there must have been someone with vision problems who passed his genes on to a significant proportion of the Japanese race. We are used to thinking in millions of people at a time, but there were easily times in the past, where countries with populations that now number in the tens of millions, had just a few thousand people in them. Everything is cyclical, and it is probable those days will come again at some time in the future. Many civilizations in the past have often collapsed at the height of their powers, often due to food problems caused by droughts, which can overwhelm any civilization very fast, and the advice in the bible about storing food from the good years to cover the lean years is something our modern politicians should certainly take into account, as world grain stocks in the last ten years have not necessarily gone in the right direction in far too many of those years. If you look at the paleontological records for North America there is even a one thousand year drought, and no civilization could cope with that. The answer when we were all nomads would have been to just walk away, but when you have planted cities then that is not an easy option.

We underestimate the vast distances that our ancestors were capable of traveling. The United States is 3,000 miles across, but if you could make just ten miles a day, then you could cover that whole distance in 300 days, and if you were foraging for food trying to walk out of a bad area, you could probably make more than ten miles a day. Obviously you can't make that distance through a dense forest, but if there is dense forest then there would be plenty of food, and you wouldn't need to move. There is an example in the past called the "Younger Dryas", which is named after an arctic plant that occurred approximately 12,800 years ago. The Younger Dryas interrupted a warming trend, and Europe was plunged rapidly into a mini ice age which lasted 1,300 years. The plunge into an ice age took place very quickly, with most of the temperature change hitting in the first year, and within less than ten years the temperature in Greenland had dropped by 27 fahrenheit (15 celsius), and that has to have caused massive disruptions. If that happened to our civilization right now, then starvations would be in the hundreds of millions, and quite possibly in the billions, and major and minor wars would break out all over the planet as people fought for food that wasn't there anymore. If you don't think that would happen, then think on this question, how long can any government keep control if more than 90% of the people haven't eaten anything in the last 48 hours? The answer is civil war, chaos, anarchy, and if food doesn't arrive quickly the collapse of civilization will follow. The Younger Dryas ended 11,500 years ago, according to the records, and it is interesting that the first civilizations that we know about arose after that event. If there had been a civilization 12,800 years ago, when the Younger Dryas started then there would be no record of it now. We think our civilization would leave signs, but if it collapsed now most of the skyscrapers in New York would fall down within 100 years, and if the sea level rose sixty feet, which is perfectly possible (and has happened in the past), then nobody would even know there had ever been a city there. Leaves and other plant debris tend to raise soil levels over time, and earlier civilizations get buried. Interstate 95 runs all the way from Miami to the Canadian border in northern Maine which is a distance of thousands of miles, but if you were looking for it in 12,000 years time what would be your chances of actually hitting it, and that's if you even thought there might be a road there. Chances are a farmer could dig down and just find pieces of broken up gravel, and think it was just assorted rocks. There is a point to this part so bear with me while I explain it at the end of the next paragraph.

One of the things that happened to the Maya before their civilization collapsed was that they suffered from several severe droughts, and it was almost certainly drought that destroyed them. Many people think the Maya vanished, but there are still about seven million Maya living in Mexico and Guatemala. Excavation at Maya burial sites shows evidence of malnutrition and a bad diet. Cost cutting and cheap food has put American civilization in a position where many people may seem as though they are adequately fed, but they are actually suffering from malnutrition because their cheap food is full of fillers and items that lack micronutrients. I will discuss this in more detail in the food and diet section, but this lack of micronutrients in both processed food, and non-processed food may well be increasing the prevalence of type 2 diabetes in the population. A small group of nomads feeding off a large area will almost always eat better than city dwellers because by their nature, cities over-farm extensive regions and pull nutrients out of the soil. I still think that the best way to farm is an area where manure from farm animals is spread over the crops, rather than fertilizer and artificial chemicals, if only because that is the way crops were naturally fertilized for the hundreds of millions of years that we have had animals, and plants on the planet. More on food in the chapter on diet.

Diet

Important Warning on Hypoglycemia (abnormally low blood sugar) for Persons Taking Insulin, Glucophage Drugs or any other Medications to Control Blood Sugar Levels

Please read the warning at the start of this book. The exercise methods and dietary methods used in this book are capable of causing significant drops in blood sugar levels. Any person reading this book who is on any kind of medication to control blood sugar must talk to his or her physician before trying any of the exercise methods or dietary methods used in this book. If you are taking any medication, do not make dietary changes or exercise changes without the assistance of a physician, as medication adjustment will be necessary to prevent excessive lowering of the blood sugar level (hypoglycemia). Hypoglycemia from using too much medication can be dangerous. Please make sure your physician reads through Appendix 1 carefully so that he or she can make note of potential large blood sugar changes in very short time periods. If you are on medication to control blood sugar I would very strongly suggest that you make walking your main exercise to reduce blood sugar levels, and that you be very careful with other forms of exercise.

We are now three to four decades away from the time that most people in America and England routinely ate healthy diets. At one time Wall Street speculated on the price of onion futures, and they did this so much that American housewives got mad. Although there are futures markets on the price of corn, wheat, and many other food products, there is now no futures market in the price of onions because American housewives had it blocked by the Onion Futures Act of 1958 after they became annoyed with Wall Street's antics. In those days there were onions in every American housewife's shopping basket, not so now. When was the last time you bought onions, carrots, potatoes or even something as simple as a radish? I'm not talking about a pre-packed mix here that may or may not be sprayed with chemicals and preservatives, I'm talking about the real thing.

Many people today eat processed food. When I was young, one of my best friends used to use the phrase "unadulterated crap" a lot, and whenever I look at a processed meal that phrase comes to mind, and so does an urge to put on a CD by the group "The Chemical Brothers". All of us know that processed food is total crap, and I cannot say this too strongly. You may think that Paris has the best scientists, and the highest knowledge in the world in the production of scents, but I am not too sure. There is another place where scents are studied, and studied, and studied, ripped apart, and chemically remade, and then remade again. That place is New Jersey, and I am talking about the food labs along the New Jersey Turnpike. They are the reason that processed food smells so much better than it tastes.

Your diet is one of the strongest tipping points that will push you into type 2 diabetes. Processed food is something you will need to give up if you want to live a decent life. Fortunately real food tastes far better than the chemical crap the food processers are giving us, and the aim of this chapter is to help you realize this, and put you in a position where you are happy preparing your own food. Before you panic and ask where you have the time to do this, let me tell you that it takes me less time to cook, and eat a meal at night than it would to drive out to a restaurant, order food, wait for it to arrive, eat it, pay for it, get back into my car and drive home, and there is one other thing, there are a lot less steps in what I do than there are in heading out for a meal.

One of the problems with restaurant food and processed food is that you have no real idea what's in it, and you also have no idea what is missing from it. In my opinion it is not so much what is in processed food that is a problem, it is the whole multitude of things that are missing from it that are a problem. Our bodies run to a large extent on enzymes that cause complex chemical reactions using very small amounts of energy. We would have a very hard time creating many of the chemicals that exist in our bodies, and even if we could create them, we would have to use prodigious amounts of energy to create chemicals and compounds that our bodies create as a matter of routine. Now all those enzymes need a supply of micronutrients coming into your body to supply the raw materials. Encoded into human DNA are the instructions to make all kinds of complex enzymes. These run much like a computer program going through various steps, and if any of the micronutrients needed to help the enzymes do their job are missing, then it is impossible to make that enzyme.

Let's take a look at uric acid because that is a chemical that builds up in our bodies. If enough uric acid builds up in your bloodstream then it can crystallize out in your joints, and the result is gout, which is incredibly painful. This is an unusual case because the instructions to make an enzyme to remove uric acid from our bodies are right there on the human genome. Unfortunately those instructions are broken on our genome, and our bodies can't make the enzyme that removes uric acid. This is caused by the fact that there is very little variation in the human genome, in fact, as I have said elsewhere, one group of seventy chimpanzees has more genetic variation than the entire seven billion humans on the planet. Gout exists solely because those instructions are broken on our DNA, which means uric acid can only be excreted slowly on days when an individual does not drink alcohol (alcohol blocks the removal of uric acid from the body) hence gout's association with heavy drinking, especially port.

Now I am talking about a problem with the instructions on our DNA here, but you can see the problems that can occur if an enzyme cannot be made. If you eat mostly processed food, then you are condemning your body to a similar situation because it lacks the raw materials to make many of the enzymes it is routinely designed to use. Over time, this is bound to cause problems. They may be minor problems or they may be major, and it is even possible that there may be a tipping point right there, in that something people used eat as part of their diets fifty years ago is now missing from our diets. You should try and eat some of your vegetables raw whenever you can. The reason for this is that many of the building blocks for enzymes are destroyed in cooking. If you are preparing vegetables for the pot, then pull one out and eat part of it. This is easier for some vegetables than others. I always use real tomatoes rather than canned tomatoes for cooking, and when I cut them up I will eat one or two of the pieces. I also do this with other vegetables whenever I can. Remember that a salad that you buy in a restaurant that has been sprayed with a chemical preservative is completely different than something you make yourself by buying the vegetables at the supermarket, and slicing them yourself. I deliberately do not want to make this book political or controversial in any way, so I am not going to attack food companies or anyone else. This book is designed solely to help you reduce the levels of sugar in your body's sugar storage reservoirs. I will point out the potential pitfalls such as processed food, and then you must navigate around them, and I will give you guidance wherever possible.

When I developed high blood sugar levels, I knew that I had to change my diet. I was in the same situation as most Americans, I was working far too hard, I was tired, and I was eating out a lot. I switched my diet very quickly and I will give you some examples of the things I ate. I also used Indian spices, and French herbs to make otherwise boring vegetables taste good. I ate a lot of vegetarian food when I was in my twenties, most of which I cooked myself, so I had a good general background in how to cook and what to do.

You should see a surge of energy within a week or two of changing your diet. Remember the situation I talked about in a previous chapter, where I heard a young man in the gym complain to the trainer that he wasn't building muscle and was tired. The trainer immediately asked him if he was getting eight hours sleep a night, and he also asked him if he was eating vegetables. Now if you go to a restaurant in America, you will find that macaroni cheese is often offered as a vegetable. This is not a vegetable, and I would also bet that the cheese sauce on the macaroni bears little resemblance to real cheese too.

I have a book by the American traveler Paul Theroux called "The Old Patagonian Express: By Train Through the Americas". In this book, Theroux decided to join the morning rush hour into Boston where his family lived, have a family reunion at Boston Central Station, and then when everyone else went to work he planned to take the train south as far as it would go (he made it to Patagonia at the end of South America). After Theroux had been on the train for a day or two, and was still heading south in the United States, he was in the dining compartment when he heard a man complaining loudly that the burger he was eating had been made using a "filler". Today we are so used to "fillers" in our food that we no longer even realize what real food is. Essentially, a filler is something that is often nutritionally useless that is cheap, and is added to food to cut costs. I have said elsewhere in this book that when cost cutting came in back in the 1980's, I said that it would destroy the West, and it has certainly destroyed Western food. I used to go to a place that made burgers in Manchester, England when I was a student. It was called "The Canadian Charcoal Pit" and it was near the university. I use their burgers as a standard for what a real burger is, and as far as I am concerned the burgers we see now in restaurants are not made like that. Either they use fillers, or they use a cheap product from the cow that can still be classed as meat, but forty years ago never made it into a burger. I don't really eat burgers very often anyway, I definitely eat less than three a year, but I know that they are not made of real food anymore, and that includes the burgers in many good restaurants too.

If you are a vegetarian and you order guacamole, then in many places in the United States what you are eating is mostly a filler, with green dye, and maybe a little bit of avocado in it. In terms of nutrition, there is whole difference between cutting into an avocado and eating it, compared with eating your green dye and filler extravaganza. Many people think that fast food is bad for you, and restaurant food is good, but that is not the case at all, it is all nutrient poor. To be fair, this is not all the restaurants' problem, we have as consumers been demanding that our food is served quickly so that we can eat it fast, and then get back to work or get back home. Often what you think has been cooked fresh has been pulled out of a freezer and microwaved, but that is our fault because we demand that the food is on our tables in less than twenty minutes, so what the restaurant does is often prepare batches in the morning, leave it sitting in the freezer, and then finish it off when somebody orders it. Meanwhile the micronutrients in the food are breaking down while it sits in the fridge. To get the best from a vegetable or fruit, it needs to be picked, and then broken by your teeth, not a knife, and those processes need to happen quickly. It needs to be chewed so that enzymes from your saliva can break it down, and then it needs to be digested by your stomach, and to get the micronutrients from the food in their best possible condition then all those things should happen within minutes of you picking the fruit or vegetable. Obviously if you wait five minutes, everything is still okay. If you wait an hour, you have lost some of the micronutrients, but you will still get most of the benefits. However, if the fruit or vegetable was picked weeks ago, as a green vegetable or fruit, and then ripened using a gas that you would never even breathe normally, then the micronutrients in it just may not be there. Remember that when the sun ripens fruit, changes happen chemically to the micronutrients that just do not happen if the fruit or vegetable was picked when it was not ripe.

Another thing to think about is travel time. I once asked a market stall holder in Long Eaton, near where I lived, how long it took him to get his fruit to market. He answered that the fruit I was buying had been landed at the docks from a ship from Spain the day before. It was put on a train from London to Birmingham (England's second largest city) overnight, and was on sale in Birmingham wholesale market at 3 am. The stallholder had driven to Birmingham during the night (50 miles or 80 kilometers), bought the fruit at 5 am, and had set up in Long Eaton by 8 am, so the fruit was on sale within 24 hours of reaching England. A supermarket cannot do that. Supermarkets have supply chains, and whatever they would like you to think, they cannot beat a market stall holder or a small corner store for speed of supply. However, they are excellent at presentation. Food often looks much better in a supermarket than on a market stall, and it often feels good because it has been preserved in some way, but at the end of the day are you buying food because it has a nice shine due to the cheap vegetable oil they sprayed it with, or are you buying food because it has a lot of micronutrients in it?

Back in the 1840s in the tenement flats for the factory workers in the UK, men would come round selling milk. There was no Trading Standards Office in those days, so often the milk was watered down by the vendors. This caused housewives to bring a hydrometer with them to put in the milk, and they could then tell whether the milk was watered down or not. We think we are sophisticated these days compared with 170 years ago, but how many people even know what a hydrometer is, and how many even know what the correct reading is for milk that hasn't been watered down. Now if only we had something like a hydrometer that we could take to the supermarket that had a reading for micronutrients on it. Can you imagine waving your special micronutrient reader above the "fresh" melon, and finding out it had two per cent of the micronutrients in it that it should have? Things would change rapidly. You would also find out that the uncut vegetables would have many more active micronutrients in them than the cut vegetables. Imagine if you pulled a processed meal out of the freezer and ran the machine over that? However, we don't have anything that can tell us this, so all I can say is this, buy real vegetables, and cut and cook them yourself if you want to eat real food. This is not as scary as you would think, in the old days your grandmother did it all the time. I will tell you what is scary though, going through the checkout and having to tell the person on the checkout what the vegetable is that you just handed him or her. On the other hand, sometimes you will be surprised. I once handed a pack of brussels sprouts to an eighteen year old, and then had a discussion with him about the best way to cook brussels sprouts (apparently his mother cooked them all the time).

When I first had high blood sugar I cooked all the food I ate at home Monday to Friday, and then at the weekend if my wife wanted to go out to eat, I went out with her. For the first eight weeks, while I lowered my blood sugar I always ordered a salad at a restaurant, and I often ate it with as little dressing as possible. Always have the dressing on the side, and one trick you can use is to run your fork through the dressing container, get salad dressing on the fork, and then run it over the salad. A woman colleague taught me that one, and it works, you will get the taste of the salad dressing without too much of it actually on your salad. Obviously with salad dressings use your common sense, if you order honey mustard dressing while you try to drop your blood sugar reservoirs then you are unlikely to be successful. After the first eight weeks, I was able to ease back a little and not be so strict about things, and there is a simple reason for that, if you have drained your blood sugar reservoirs then you have some leeway, whereas if they are full to the brim then even looking at a honey mustard dressing is likely to push you over the edge. Okay, I was joking there, but here is an interesting point, as soon as you think about eating a meal your pancreas begins to push insulin into your body ahead of time.

In those first eight weeks I had to eat out at lunchtime. What I did was to eat out at a Southern Barbecue restaurant. Now most of you will immediately think "loaded with sugar" and calories" when I use the phrase "Southern Barbecue", but what I ordered was a meal which was basically a green leaf salad with meat in it. This is the perfect kind of meal if you are trying to lower blood sugar because greens, such as lettuce, are a complex carbohydrate with a lot of fiber. Complex carbohydrates break down slowly, and your body has to work hard to remove sugars from them so you get a double benefit. Firstly, the lettuce and salad greens have very little impact on your blood sugar, and secondly, your body has to use more energy to break them down than if you ate a simple carbohydrate like a cookie. In the first eight week period do not have any sauces at all, as many of those will be loaded with sugar, even the ones that supposedly are non-sweet. Also be wary of artificial sweeteners because some of them break down into some really nasty substances in your liver, and one of the things you need to do if you are to free yourself from type 2 diabetes is to take more care of your liver.

I just took a quick exercise break after the last paragraph, and one thing occurred to me while I was walking backwards and forwards from one end of the house to the other, and this is important. I live pretty much a normal life in terms of food. If I go to Barnes and Noble, I will have a cinnamon scone or whatever I want, from their café. I don't eat their cheesecake much because it tastes too sweet, and I suspect their stuff is loaded with sugar. Now if I went to Barnes and Noble every day, then I wouldn't do this, but if I am there at the weekend I usually just have something. I rarely have two things, in fact that almost never happens unless we are there a long time, but why would you need two snacks? I usually take a packet of peanuts or cashew nuts with me, and if I want something else then that is what I have. I never have any of the flavored coffees that are loaded with sugar because that is just a waste of calories, in my opinion. I drink green tea or occasionally coffee while I am there, and I never have flavored coffee.

One reason I can eat what I want most of the time is that I take a lot of exercise. Remember the example from Czarist Russia where the Russian army used to attack from five sides at once. Well this is a flexible program, and because a strong part of my attack on type 2 diabetes is on the exercise front, then I have a little more flexibility on the food front. If you take less exercise, then you might have to be stricter with what you eat, but at the end of the day, it is up to you how you do this once you have your blood sugar lowered. My standard routine is to exercise five days a week, and take two days off. This suits me. I am not a believer in exercising for just three days a week because if you look at what our ancestors did, then it is unlikely they chased game, and foraged for just three days a week, and then sat around doing no exercise for the other four days.

One thing I did notice when I started to get organized with taking blood sugar readings, was that my blood sugar reading on a Monday morning was often higher than on a Tuesday morning, and that had to be due to either exercising less or eating out at the weekend. I know I am repeating myself here because I have said this elsewhere in the book, but numbers like this or trends like this are really important to note in the early days when you are trying to drop your blood sugar.

There is much to be said for eating a vegetable or a fruit within minutes of having picked it. One time when I was in my twenties, I stayed with one of my friends and his wife. When it was time to cook the vegetables, Juliet sent John out into the garden to pull up some carrots. Five minutes after the carrots were pulled they were in the pot, and half an hour after that we were eating them. I have never eaten carrots that tasted like that. I remember as a boy aged seven, going to the house of relatives in Carlisle, England and being given fresh peas out of a pod. I only ate the peas because my elder cousins were eating them, but they just tasted completely different than anything my mother gave me.

Herbs are very easy to grow, unless you live somewhere really cold. France has a perfect climate for growing herbs, and many French people just stroll into their gardens, and pick the herbs minutes before putting them into the pan. Fresh basil in your cooking tastes great, and if it is warm enough where you live, basil is really easy to grow. Herbs do well in container pots if you don't have good soil where you live. Even if you live in an apartment you can grow a few things on your balcony if the rules permit.

Americans are always surprised when I tell them how many things just won't grow in England. Even though the winters are incredibly cold in New England, they can grow many more things there in the summer than can be grown in England. The main problem with England is cloudiness and lack of sunlight. Annapolis in Maryland actually has ten inches more rain than Nottingham where I lived in the UK, but a lot of the annual rainfall in Annapolis comes down in heavy storms, whereas the UK specializes in Seattle style drizzle. I remember one vacation in Wales with my first girlfriend where it rained every single day, all day, for the first ten days of the holiday. She was staying at a hotel with her parents, and I was staying at a campsite in a tent nearby. Liz was not bothered by the rain, and we sat on the beach all day reading books under umbrellas, which was actually quite fun. The rain was windswept, and every night for the first few days I had to bail my tent out with a cup where the rain got in, although it didn't make it to my sleeping bag. The tent was waterproof, but the rain was coming in through the zipper. I was just 18 years old, and in a one man tent. One of the other campers saw me baling the tent out, and gave me some clear plastic sheeting that I could put over the zipper and that stopped it.

I used to walk up to the hotel every morning after eating breakfast, and spend the day with my girlfriend and her family. The fresh air, and walking in the Welsh hills was really healthy, and I came back from that vacation very fit. I don't think my girlfriend's father really wanted me along. I had to make my own way down to Wales because their car was full with luggage, but to be fair he was very protective of his daughter, and was very much of the old school and had not moved with the times. My girlfriend was very insistent I went down there though so I went, and it gave me a real appreciation of the Gower Peninsula, which is to the west of the City of Swansea in South Wales. In those days there was almost nobody on the beaches down there, and it was incredibly unspoilt. I have no idea what it is like now. Although we had ten days of Welsh rain, the last four days were clear blue sky days, and days like that in Wales really show what a beautiful country it is.

When I moved to Alaska in 1997 I was exposed to massive portions in American restaurants for the first time. Many immigrants to this country put on weight due to the portion sizes, and that was something I had to fight against. All food is flown into Alaska, and fresh vegetables are very expensive with tomatoes being a dollar each (and you thought it was expensive where you live). I tried growing tomatoes on the front porch in Eagle River where it was sunny, and had no problem getting them to grow but only one of them ripened. If I still lived there, I would probably have a greenhouse and grow things. Many people blame portion size for weight gain in America, but weight gain is going on all over the world now, except possibly areas of Asia where they speak tonal languages. Even Bollywood film stars are fighting their weight now, whereas their parents' generation didn't have to worry so much about it.

When I started working on getting my blood sugar down, I quickly focused on very simple food. I had been eating out with the family quite a bit at night, but I stopped that during the week and only ate out at weekends. I am going to tell you exactly what I ate, rather than giving you general advice because there may be something there that tipped the balance into lowering my blood sugar. At night I settled fairly quickly into eating frozen salmon and brussels sprouts. Publix supermarkets near us had some very good brussels sprouts from Mexico, which were much bigger than the ones I see in the United States and bigger than the ones in England. I did this because I was monitoring my blood sugar every morning, and I noticed that it was lower when I ate leafy greens than when I ate canned tomatoes with fish. There is more detail on blood sugar numbers in the chapter on "Climbing out of Diabetes" and in Appendix 1, but my morning blood sugar after eating leafy greens and fish the night before, was 10 to 20 points lower than my blood sugar when eating canned tomatoes and fish. This was very likely the point at which I realized that all processed foods had to be gone from my diet. I prepared the fish by just straight boiling it in water. Obviously there are tastier ways to eat fish than this, but my aim was to reduce my blood sugar, and at that point that was all that mattered because I really didn't want to go on metformin. I still do not take any drugs to control blood sugar.

Now you may wish to vary things, and eat meat instead of fish and that is fine, I am just telling you what I ate. If you eat meat, do not eat sauces with it because you never know what is in them. Your diet may be a little bland during the first eight weeks while you attack your blood sugar levels, but at the end of the day your blood sugar levels have to come first, not your taste buds. I have probably said this elsewhere before; we have all become conditioned that every meal should be a good meal. Unless you are French, or live in a French speaking area, forget that because in Anglo-Saxon countries food typically sustained life rather than gave pleasure. This has resulted, in America at least, of a tradition of sauces loaded with sugar to improve the flavor of meat, which is not a good habit to be in. We have to remember also that some American eating habits grew up out of a necessity to put as much weight on a child as necessary because of high mortality rates among children in the seventeenth, and eighteenth centuries, and adding sugar was a good way to get calories into a child.

I cannot stress how vitally important it is to give up sugar in the first eight weeks. I told you in chapter one how I gave up eating sugar for five years when I was twelve years old, and if a twelve year old boy can do it, then you can do it. It has never bothered me if people are eating things around me that I'm not eating, but you may be different in that respect. If that is the case then talk to your family and friends, and ask them to be careful around you. Remember that sometimes people around you secretly want to sabotage you, whether consciously or unconsciously, so be on the lookout for that. If anyone starts telling you it is okay to eat something that you don't want to eat, then walk away in mid conversation if you have to.

There may be some overlap between this section and the section called "Climbing out of Diabetes", but I want to make sure that you know exactly what I ate. There will be more detail, and more quoting of blood sugar numbers in the other section. At weekends when we went out to eat, I ate salads for probably at least the first six months. I may not have needed to do that, it just felt healthy. Usually the salad had meat in, and there was a place on Jacksonville Beach called the Crab Shack that did a great Cobb Salad, and my wife and I would sit on the elevated back deck and eat looking out over the water, which was really nice. With meals out, all I drank was water as it was a safe, easy option.

For breakfast every day I ate General Mills Fiber One cereal, which is now known as Fiber One Original. I had been advised by my doctor to eat more fiber. I don't eat that now, although I may give it a try again. Most of the carbohydrates in that cereal are insoluble fiber, and it was not sweetened with sugar. I would have had 2% milk or vitamin D milk on it (if you are in the UK or Australia then vitamin D milk in the United States is ordinary milk - pretty much all milk in the US is homogenized). The fat in the milk will slow down the absorption of carbohydrates, and it is possible I used vitamin D milk for the first eight weeks for that reason. If you use soy milk instead of real milk then things will work differently so be aware of that.

I think that covers what I ate. I knew how to cook, which put me at a distinct advantage and made it easier for me. Most people like broccoli, so if you prefer that instead of brussels sprouts then you may want to try that. Remember that broccoli is actually a flower, not a leafy green (check your gardening book), but the main point of using leafy greens is that they are very low in carbs, and I am sure that applies to broccoli too. Some medications, like blood thinners, react badly to leafy greens, so be wary of that. As always, check with your doctor before changing your diet. Also, ease in any changes to diet slowly, rather than changing everything at once, in case it upsets your stomach. Some of what I ate in the first eight weeks was bland, but I was aiming to reduce blood sugar, not have a pleasant dining experience, and going to restaurants that use the phrase "dining experience" in their adverts may well be what has gotten some people into trouble with type 2 diabetes in the first place.

I don't eat pizza. I don't see any nutritional value in pizza at all, and it will dump carbs into your body like crazy. Every time gas prices go above $3.50 in Florida, the economy slows down, people stop going out and restaurants start going bust. I have seen all kinds of restaurants go out of business in the Jacksonville area since 2008, and when I went to Daytona Beach which is a real tourist area, there were shut down restaurants all over the place, but I have never seen a restaurant that serves pizza shut down, even in the depths of the recession. This might well be one reason why type 2 diabetes is so high in the United States. I don't go as far as to refuse pizza if it is offered to me at somebody's house, but I don't seek it out.

I eat brown rice, but I don't eat pasta and I definitely don't eat white rice. An Indian once told me that Indians have very high triglycerides due to all the white basmati rice they eat. The American medical profession includes brown rice with white rice, but brown rice breaks down much more slowly in the body. Chinese medicine says that it is okay for people with type 2 diabetes to eat brown rice. When I use the term brown rice, I do not mean "easy cook brown rice" that is ready in ten minutes. That falls under the classification of processed food, and I don't know what they do to it. I have a lot of experience of eating beans, and the carbs from beans are more along the lines of complex carbohydrates and push sugar into you more slowly. Obviously you want to avoid anything that puts sugar into you fast. Cooked carrots can do that, but a raw grated carrot is a whole different ball game and will give you a lot of fiber. Again, do not use ready peeled carrots in cooking because I don't know whether they are sprayed with anything to stop them going off. Peeling a carrot takes only a minute, especially if you use the right kind of peeler. Some people reading this will have very little experience of peeling vegetables. The best kind of vegetable peeler is one with a rotating head, and I can peel very fast with this one. I am telling you this because it is important to make things as easy as possible if you are about to start cooking for yourself.

I eat a lot of beans and lentils. I learnt how to cook beans when I was in my twenties. Some people worry about gas with beans so here are a few pointers. A lot of what causes gas from the beans is in the cooking water. If you buy canned beans throw away the water, wash them thoroughly in a colander, and then add them to whatever you are cooking. A quick and easy recipe with beans is to fry three or four onions in olive oil, and when the onions are cooked add the drained and washed beans to the pan. The beans will absorb the oil and dry the pan out very fast, so just stir them into the onions for a minute or two and then turn the heat off. One can of beans and three or four onions will make one person enough for two meals. This will do as a quick lunch on a weekend. I do this with pinto beans. The beans I prefer are 365 beans from Whole

Foods. I have tried several different varieties. All that is in the canned beans should be water and salt, although when I used to cook dried beans I did not add salt.

If you are cooking dried beans then boil them for ten minutes and then change the water, which gets rid of a lot of the starches that cause gas because they are already out in the cooking water at that point. Use a stainless steel colander with hot water, I don't trust plastics with hot water, and plastic molecules can bind to organic molecules if they get into your system. Try as many different kinds of beans as you can. Years ago there was a jazz café in Glastonbury in the UK called "The Blue Note Café", which was run by an American, and his bean soup was incredible. Unfortunately he moved on, and I don't know where he is now.

I used to go to Glastonbury quite a lot at one time, and we used to sit and drink coffee in the Blue Note Café and talk for hours. Quite a few of us used to go down, and I remember the first time I went down there were twenty-eight of us camping. I was in a tent with my friend Mike and his roommate Debbie, who was not Mike's partner, but lived with a guy called Damien who was also a roommate of Mike's. Nathan was two or three at the time and he was with my parents for the weekend. Having a young child meant I was conditioned to wake at 6:30 am, and Mike and Debbie slept on. I went and showered, and they were still asleep so I walked into Glastonbury. As I walked into the town, there was a man in his twenties with long hair walking along playing a guitar, and he was actually really good and that just made the whole weekend for me.

One time I went to Glastonbury we stayed at a bed and breakfast owned by the widow of a British diplomat. She had grown up in Glastonbury and she told me she lived there when Dion Fortune lived there. She said they could see the lights as Dion and her group went up to Glastonbury Tor in the middle of the night. Her exact comment to me was that in those days everyone thought Dion Fortune and her group were a bunch of nutcases, and now the whole town is built around her. That was a really interesting comment. I am reading a book by Dion Fortune at the moment called "The Sea Priestess" and it is actually quite good. The world described in this book is pretty much the same time period as the British television show "Downton Abbey" if you have seen that, and is a million miles from the world of today.

There used to be a sign at the bottom of Glastonbury Tor, which doesn't seem to be there anymore which was quite interesting. The sign stated that on November 15, 1539 King Henry VIII hanged Richard Whiting, the Abbott of Glastonbury Abbey, at the base of the Tor. Although Henry VIII is badly painted in history, America only exists as an English speaking country because Henry VIII stole all the money from the Catholic Church. Before that he was relatively broke, after he robbed the church he was able to build huge battle cruisers. In fact, one of the ships Henry VIII built was so overloaded with cannons that it sank when it was launched, and it was only raised towards the end of the twentieth century. The skeletons of the sailors who went down with the ship were still on board when they raised it.

Grains were never part of the diet of our ancestors until agriculture was developed. Grains will dump sugar into your bloodstream very quickly, and since the best way to fatten cows is to fill them full of corn, then it may not be a good idea to eat too many grains. They should certainly not be as big a part of your diet as the American government food pyramid suggests. One of the interesting things I read recently is that in areas of the world where grains are not consumed, schizophrenia is almost non-existent. This was being studied in the early 1980s, and may have been a casualty of the Reagan budget cuts. This begs further research, and two questions spring immediately to mind. The first question is whether a grain free diet could prevent schizophrenia, and the second is, would a grain free diet cure schizophrenia if somebody had it? Then there is another very important question. If consumption of grains makes a small proportion of the population completely insane, does it make the rest of the population slightly insane? Maybe nomads are normal, and the rest of us are all slightly off our rockers. Just the thought of that is quite amusing, and considering some of the things that have been done in the name of civilization, it is also quite possible. Another point that springs to mind is the low tolerance of native groups to alcohol, and their seeming addiction to it. Almost all alcohol is brewed from grain. What if it is not the alcohol that is causing the problems for native groups, but exposure to chemicals in grain? These are just a few thoughts, but this really should be investigated. We should take a group of supposedly sane, rational Europeans or Americans, and take them off grains for a year. If they got withdrawal symptoms a day or two after the grains were removed, then that really would be interesting. A lot of the studies appear to have been done by F.C. Dohan. Here are two links at the US National Library of Medicine:

Is schizophrenia rare if grain is rare?

http://www.ncbi.nlm.nih.gov/pubmed/6609726

Reports by F.C. Dohan:

http://www.ncbi.nlm.nih.gov/pubmed?term=Dohan%20FC%5BAuthor%5D&cauthor=true&cauthor_uid=6609726

I am going to give you a few basic recipes that will get you started cooking your own food if you have no experience of cooking. Many people reading this book will be excellent cooks, but others may not, and I don't want to advise you to give up processed food, and then leave you floundering with nothing to eat. There is a great book by Tosca Reno called "The Eat-Clean Diet". I have had this for a few years, and there are some very good recipes in it. If I remember correctly, Tosca Reno designed the recipes so that they did not dump a lot of carbs quickly into the body, although the main focus of the book was to eat healthy food. There are a lot more recipes in that book than I could ever give you, and I strongly recommend buying it. When I bought it back in 2008 there was only one version of the book, but now there are multiple versions, including one written specifically for men in collaboration with her late husband, Robert Kennedy who is mentioned in the exercise chapter of this book. I specifically remember cooking one recipe in the book which used zucchinis in an omelet that my family really liked, and I would never have thought of putting zucchinis in an omelet (zucchinis are called courgettes in the UK). If you buy Tosca's book, then you will never be short of good healthy recipes to cook.

If you are cooking vegetables that are bland, then it may well be worth buying an Indian cookbook too because the Indians are experts at making otherwise bland vegetables taste really good. A can of lentil soup in England is one of the blandest things you can ever eat, with the only flavoring pretty much being salt from what I remember, but an Indian lentil curry is a whole different ball game. I will include a recipe for lentil curry below. Again, these recipes are just to get you started, I expect you to take them, experiment with them, and then make them your own. You may prefer more cumin, coriander, curry powder, or turmeric than I would. In England, when I grew up curry powder had a kind of negative image, but if you look at what is actually in curry powder by reading the ingredients on the back, then you will see that it has some really good spices in. Garlic is also a great ingredient. American garlic is not as strong as English garlic, and does not have the same effect on your breath the next day as English garlic does. I once grew garlic in a container pot using some cloves from garlic that I bought in a supermarket. I used the green shoots from the top of the garlic to add flavor in cooking and they were like a very strong version of chives.

The three recipes below are vegetable soup, meat stew, and lentil curry. I do not claim to be an expert cook, but if you have very little experience of cooking then these may get you started. They are all made with fresh ingredients from the supermarket and use Indian spices, garlic, and European herbs for flavoring. If you are already a really experienced cook, then look at the ingredients not the recipes, and design your own recipes using similar ingredients. Any one of these recipes will be far better for you than eating out at a restaurant, and once you get used to not having hidden, added sugar and fat in your food, then you will likely find that you really like the flavors of natural food. None of the ingredients are expensive, and you can find all of them at your local supermarket. Sometimes the food in the Mexican section of your supermarket may be priced cheaper than the food in the American section, especially with things like lentils and beans. If the supermarket has its own brand of lentils then buy those, there really is no difference from the major brands. Avoid lentils with packs of spices with them unless you can be absolutely sure that they have no added sugar or fat in them. Remember that anything made from corn will dump added carbs right into your system and raise your blood sugar, and some of the spice packs have ingredients like that in them. Corn is heavily subsidized by the United States government, which is one of the main reasons why it is in everything. Corn is even being added to some yogurts now. Remember that if you don't cook the food yourself, and add all the ingredients yourself then you really have no idea what the heck is in there.

It is also worth trying unusual things. I eat Korean seaweed that I buy in Whole Foods. I do that because it has micronutrients in it that you just don't see in your normal diet. Mushrooms are something you can add to food that have no carbs in them. Although nuts have a bad rap for having a lot of calories in them, they do have nutrients in that we do not often see in our normal food. Don't just try the standard nuts like peanuts and cashews, try some different types and also, if you have the time, try buying nuts in their shells and shelling them. In England when I was growing up, people always bought nuts at Christmas and it was always fun sitting in front of the fire and shelling them. In England in the 1990s, everyone was pretty much off work from December 24th to January 2nd, so it was a really nice long holiday, and a time for total relaxation. One other thing, a 50 cents packet of peanuts as a snack may well stop you buying that piece of cake, or other carb loaded processed food when you are hungry.

Recipes

The recipes below are just recipes to get you started, vegetable soup, meat stew, and lentil curry.

Vegetable Soup

4 carrots
2 onions
1 to 2 zucchinis (courgettes in the UK)
3 to 4 tomatoes depending on size (fresh, not canned)
Garlic
1 can of pinto beans (or your preferred bean)

Cumin
Coriander
Turmeric
Herbs de Provence
Basil leaves, or dried basil
Rosemary
Oregano
Tarragon
Thyme
1 to 2 tablespoons of Italian cold pressed olive oil (optional)

Peel and chop the carrots, onions, zucchini, and tomatoes and put them in a medium size pan. Add enough water to cover the vegetables then add the herbs and spices. I usually just shake the spices in and alter it for taste as I cook. I would say add 1 teaspoon of cumin, 1 to 2 teaspoons of coriander, and 1 flat teaspoon of turmeric. If you wish you can also add mild curry powder, although I don't do this so it is not in the list. Bring it to the boil, and if you want to add olive oil then pour it onto a spoon and add it when the water is fairly hot, but not boiling. That way the oil will just run off the tablespoon when you put it in the water and not stick to it. I usually cook it for 25 minutes and I add the pinto beans about five minutes before I take it off. This will depend on how you like your vegetables. It is important to pour the water off the canned beans, and wash them in a colander. As I said above, I use 365 pinto beans from whole foods. You can use any of these herbs listed, if you are missing one it doesn't matter. If you have a herb you like using then try it. This recipe is just a guide to get you started. Experiment and enjoy. Preparation time should be 10 to 15 minutes, cooking time should be a maximum of half an hour, so you should be sitting down to eat in less than an hour. While it cooks you are free to do something else. As long as there is enough water in the pan it won't burn and it won't stick.

I used to eat this with salmon or with brown rice. Brown rice will take about forty minutes to cook, so when I do it I put the rice on first. I have experimented with rice cookers, but pans are much easier to clean than rice cookers. The first time I went into a store in England and asked to buy a rice cooker, the store clerk looked at me as though I was insane and refused to believe such things existed. This was in summer 1990, now you can buy them anywhere. The first practical electric rice cooker was invented by a Japanese man, Yoshitada Minami, just after World War II.

Meat Stew

1 to 2 pounds of stewing beef
4 to 6 carrots (use real carrots, not ready peeled carrots)
4 to 6 potatoes (in the US red russets seem to be best although it varies with the season)
3 to 4 tomatoes, depending on size, use fresh not canned. These are optional.
In winter, add seasonal vegetables such as rutabaga (swede in the UK), parsnips and turnips
Garlic 1 to 3 cloves (optional)
Cumin
Coriander
Turmeric
Herbs de Provence
Basil leaves or dried basil
Rosemary
Tarragon
Thyme

Use a large pan for this recipe. The meat used in this recipe is a cheap cut of meat but it will go far for the price, which is why I use it. I boil the meat for one and a half hours before adding the vegetables although an hour is fine if you wish to do it quicker – the meat will be softer if you cook it longer. Wash the meat under the faucet, and watch it while you bring it to the boil, which will take about five minutes. You add all the herbs, spices, and garlic at the start after you have covered the meat with water.

When it boils you need to be standing there ready to turn the heat down, or the water will boil right over the top due to the juices from the meat. The cooks reading this book will already know that, but some people reading this book will be inexperienced cooks, so I am stating everything that needs to be done. I was once in Wal-Mart, which is a place I never ever shop at nowadays, and I heard a young woman say to her partner that she was going to select something to cook for that evening's dinner. I then watched in disbelief as she pulled a microwaveable freezer meal off the shelf. That is not cooking, but there may be some people who have very little experience of cooking reading this, and I do not want anybody to be discouraged because I didn't state something that they needed to know to cook this. On our cooker, which is electric, I turn the heat down to 7 after it boils, and keep it boiling slowly. I have found the meat cooks through better with the top off the pan, although you can put the lid on if you want and simmer it.

You will need to keep an eye on it and add water while it cooks, as the water level will fall. After an hour and a half add the vegetables, and then cook for approximately 20 to 25 minutes. At that point pull some of the stew out and put it in a bowl. Let it cool and make sure the vegetables are cooked to your liking. If you are not used to cooking, you will get a good feel for this after cooking it a few times.

Lentil Curry

One pound (454 grams) of dried red lentils, or brown lentils, washed and cleaned
Mild curry powder - or stronger if you wish – if you are not used to curry powder or spicy (hot in the UK) foods then start with 1 flat teaspoon of mild curry powder. If you are used to curry powder then use more.
Coriander 1 to 2 heaped teaspoons
Cumin 1 heaped teaspoon
Turmeric 1 flat teaspoon
1 carrot grated
1 onion cut, or chopped finely
3 to 4 tomatoes cut into small pieces

Wash the lentils first and then add them to the pan. Use a large pan. Add all the ingredients to the pan and cover with water. Bring to boil and then boil for 40 minutes. Add additional water as needed through the cooking process. After 40 minutes the lentils should be ready, but taste them to make sure. When they are ready, take the pan off the heat, let it cool a little, and then mash the lentils with a potato masher. Serve with brown rice, pita bread, or Indian naan bread. You can also use this as a side dish with meat if you wish. Again this recipe is just a guide, experiment with the ingredients. You can add more coriander and curry powder if you wish. Be careful with adding too much cumin or turmeric as that can ruin the taste. If it tastes bland, then add more coriander and curry powder, and possibly a little more cumin or use extra garlic next time. If you cook this several times you should be able to experiment and get a really good flavor. I first learnt the basics of this recipe from my brother-in-law, Tony Pinchess, who was an incredible cook even by the time I first met him when we were both twenty-one years old.

A Note on the Recipes

I am not an expert cook so these recipes are just to get you started if you have no real experience of cooking. If cooked properly they can taste far better than any processed food. They are designed to be healthy and are not designed to be extremely low carb, but having said that, they will have less carbs in than many restaurant meals or processed packaged meals. Experiment and enjoy cooking them. We are all busy and short of time these days, so these recipes are all designed to give you time to walk away and just leave them to cook, while you get on with something else. Once I have brought something to the boil, then I am usually exercising in the gym, or writing on my computer and I just use a timer to make sure I check back in at the appropriate times.

Diet and the Liver

I said in the introduction that one way researchers give lab rats type 2 diabetes is to give them high doses of fructose. This leads to a fatty liver, and after that, type 2 diabetes follows. You can look at the liver two ways. In one version, the liver is an incredible filter that breaks down the food you put in your body and removes any toxins. In the other version, the liver is a dumping ground for all the crap we put into our bodies, which rapidly becomes clogged from overuse. My grandfather (the one who went to World War I as a fourteen or fifteen year old) used to grow all kinds of things in his garden. One of the things he would grow was strawberries. Strawberries that are fresh from the garden, and picked only when they have been ripened by the sun taste incredible, and real fresh fruit beats any kind of artificial flavor in the foods we have now. If I eat strawberries from a garden, then when the food is broken down in my liver all it has to deal with are the kind of things human livers have been used to dealing with for millions of years, and if you go back through our primate ancestors then this runs into tens of millions of years. That means the liver is well adapted to dealing with normal strawberries. Now suppose I eat something that has strawberry flavoring in. The correct chemical name for one type of strawberry flavoring is "ethyl methylphenylglycidate".

Now let me be absolutely, and totally clear here. I am just giving you information. All food processes in the United States are evaluated by the FDA, which means everything in food in the United States is safe. Demand from consumers to produce food as cheaply as possible likely means that it is impossible to produce strawberry flavoring by boiling up millions of tons of strawberries, and condensing the resultant product down into flavoring. I just prefer to eat food that I have prepared myself. The flavors in all the foods I prepare come from herbs, spices, and the food itself. That is not the same as having my own land, being a farmer, and growing all my own food myself, but it is closer than buying processed food.

I remember going to the house of friends in Alaska for dinner. The family we went to see lived on a lake, and often had parties in the winter with bonfires on the ice. That time there was just them and our family, and Judy had cooked a meal that was very simple but also incredibly healthy, and comprised meat, potatoes, and various vegetables. That was one of the healthiest meals I ate in Alaska. Most significant was that neither Judy nor her husband Phil was overweight, they both looked very healthy, and I believe that they ate like that all the time. I probably eat a lot like that now but I didn't at the time.

Let's go back to the Vikings, and look at the kind of foods they ate. The Vikings that invaded and settled in Scotland came mainly from Norway. Most of them came from settlements in fjords, and in fact, the word fjord is a Scandinavian word. The Gulf Stream flows onto the Norwegian coast, and despite its high latitude, a good part of the Norwegian coast is ice fee all year. One thousand years ago the fjords had abundant fish in them, and that made up a good part of the protein in the diet of the Vikings. One of the things I noticed in Alaska was the huge numbers of wild animals, especially bears. Bears live according to very definite natural cycles. They hibernate all winter and produce their young in the spring. The late summer, and fall, is based around putting as much weight on as possible to get ready for the long winter. In Alaska, as well as in northern Europe, fruit appears in the fall and bears that don't have access to fish eat as many berries as they can to put their winter weight on. Bears that live by a river with abundant fish, especially salmon, typically weigh a lot more than bears that don't. This makes me wonder if people who are originally of north European stock should be eating fruit all the year round, or whether we are naturally evolved to eat fruit only in the fall. This is just a thought, but it maybe it needs some thinking about, especially given the fact that bears in Alaska use fruit to put as much weight on as possible for winter.

Summary on the Diet Section

I would have liked to have said a lot more in the section on the liver than I did. Last night I was doing extensive reading in a book I have on Chinese medicine, and a doubt crept in about something that was in that book, so I have decided not to include some things in this book that I was originally going to include. I am also a little wary of inadvertently making a comment that may be regarded as critical about any kind of food company, so I erased a good part of what I had written, partly because although I know quite a lot about certain things, I do not have the advanced knowledge of chemistry that I really need here.

Suffice to say that I feel the liver is a key part of the fight against type 2 diabetes. There are instructions on our DNA to make all kinds of enzymes, and there are three fields where I feel science in the twenty first century has lagged behind where it should be.

One is the study of enzymes, I feel we are at least 100 years behind where we should be. The second is the study of sound waves, especially high frequency sound waves. I told you earlier about my computer science professor, who was able to make steel bus stops wave about in the air with just a tuning fork. The third is the study of catalysts, and again we may well be 100 years behind where we should be in this area. The instructions to make enzymes on our DNA work sequentially like a computer program until all the steps are done, and then the process switches off and the enzyme is ready. Suppose your body is making an enzyme that needs 20 steps to be produced. The process fails at step 18 because an essential micronutrient is missing. That micronutrient would have been there in your grandfather, but because you eat pizza, instead of some of the things your grandfather ate, one micronutrient is missing. You now have a partially made enzyme. That partially made enzyme has to be trucked back to the liver and dismantled. But what if the liver is not geared up for this dismantling because none of the last 5,000 generations of humans have ever had production of this enzyme fail? Stress is then put on the liver as it dismantles the broken enzyme. Another possibility is that the partially made enzyme never makes it to the liver, and binds onto something it shouldn't be attached to, causing cell death. Again, that has to be corrected. I told you earlier in the book, about the medical professor who had a request from his students for young cadavers, instead of older ones. The young American cadavers were in excellent physical health, but their livers were the livers of old men and women even though they were just in their twenties. Did their livers have type 2 diabetes time bombs sitting in them because they had been put under stress and damaged? We don't know that, I can only put this out as a question, but what I will say to you is this; please find out as much as you can about your livers. With all the additives and chemicals in food, we are no doubt stressing our livers out. I read a book on the liver by a doctor called Sandra Cabot, and she mentioned a case where she had worked to repair the liver of a young man who had never consumed alcohol but ate pepperoni pizza almost every day. I have known a few people in their twenties with irritable bowel syndrome. One thing they all had in common was a diet of pizza and beer.

Something has changed in our diet that is responsible in some way for this outbreak of type 2 diabetes. It happens with thin people, as well as overweight people. It could just as easily be a micronutrient that we are not eating, as well as something that is new in our diet. I would actually put my money on the solution being something that is missing from our diets, rather than on something bad that is in our diets. When I eat out at a restaurant, whether it is a fast food restaurant, or a "normal" restaurant, I am often hungry within one hour of eating. There is absolutely no way I should be hungry within one hour of eating. If I cook for myself, I am never hungry within one hour of eating, it just doesn't happen and also I eat less when I cook for myself than I do in a restaurant. That just seems odd to me.

In conclusion, I don't believe you can ever beat type 2 diabetes if you continue to eat a lot of processed food. You don't have to stop right now this second, but make tomorrow, or the next day, a day that is free of all processed food. Then do the same thing two days later. Use the starter recipes I have given you and order Tosca Reno's book from Amazon, it will be here in a few days. The key to cooking for yourself, is ease of work. If it takes you two hours to prepare, then you might only do it once. I try to do all the work up front, and then cook whatever I am cooking in a pan on the stove, just using a timer. While it cooks, I do something else. That may be the exercise room, I might go on the computer and write, or I might read a book. The key thing is that the food is cooking itself, without me needing to stand over it. Even with the meat stew recipe, I might just have to check that once every half hour, and that check might take one minute to make sure there is enough water in it. At the weekends, maybe I spend more time, but at night I need something that is not too taxing in terms of effort when I get home from work. I cook immediately I arrive home, and then it is done and out of the way. I eat the food when it is ready, put some away for the next day, and then go and exercise.

Remember also, the first eight weeks while you attack your body's sugar reserves, will take more effort than the maintenance role you will play for most of the time. Eat complex carbohydrates as much as you can. You can relax a little once you have your blood sugar reservoirs down, and you will see that in your numbers. I have come to like grated carrots, and I eat those a lot.

Stir fries of things like green peppers, onions, mushrooms, and tomatoes can be really nice, and will usually make extra. Cut the vegetables yourself, and do not buy them ready made. Remember the things our grandmothers said not to eat too much of, things like pasta and bread. I have said elsewhere, my father used to have a slice of buttered bread with his meal at night. I tried that one time and I found I started to put weight on, so I stopped it. The saying "you are what you eat" has a lot of truth in it.

Relaxation, Meditation and Lucid Dreaming

This may seem like an odd title, but you would be surprised how relaxed a really intense dream can make you. My sister and my son both dream every night and always have, but when I was young I never remembered any of my dreams. When I was in my twenties I taught myself how to dream, and I experimented with flying dreams, falling dreams and also dream control, which can take you to a whole different level. The sense of relaxation attained from a good lucid dream (lucid means a dream that is real, in full color and seems like you are really there) can be amazing, and if you have never had a lucid dream but you suffer a lot from stress, then read on. Stress can really chip away at your body's blood sugar control, and stress is a definite tipping point. By the way, if you hit bottom in a falling dream you don't die at all or I would have been dead tens of times over. Falling dreams are closely related to flying dreams, and if you practice flying dreams like I did, then you will hit bottom now and then. Hitting the ground in a flying dream is not even scary, so that is one old myth demolished. Here is an example of a flying dream I generated after becoming partially aware in a dream:

I became aware that I was dreaming, and a part of my mind remembered that I was aiming to produce a flying dream. To do that, I needed something to fly off. Green grass appeared in front of me, and ahead of the green grass a cliff top appeared. The green of the grass was incredible, and way stronger than green in real life. In an instant I accelerated down the grass towards the cliff edge and flew off it, and then I was flying. The feeling was intense and exhilarating.

This is another example of something I used to do all the time, such as yoga or certain exercises. It really is that easy to produce and control a dream. Dreams like this make you feel good during the day, and you wake up more refreshed if you have had a lucid dream than with normal sleep. I have no idea how to interpret dreams, and I'm not even sure I believe in the interpretation of dreams, but I do know a lot about how to create, and control, a dream. If you are interested in this part then read on because it can certainly help you to relax.

When I was young, I hardly ever dreamed. I remember when I was very young, I used to lie in bed and imagine I was running down an airport runway, the kind they used for small propeller planes. I would run faster, and faster, and then I would take off. After that, I would go and help people. I remember doing that a lot when I was young. You may say, how can a three or four year old boy help people, but if you are in a dream, are you really three or four years old? Also what is in control when you are asleep? Is your subconscious a small three or four year old boy, or is it something ancient with infinite wisdom? Whatever the answer to that is, it was important to me to go and help people. I have no idea what happened after I fell asleep, but I do know that my intention on running down that imaginary runway and taking off, was to go and help people. Before I went to school, I never needed much sleep. I had a clock in my room and I would lie awake until 10:30 pm, and then I would go to sleep. I woke every morning at 4:30 am, and I would lie there in bed until my parents came to wake me up. I was probably about four years old when I had those memories. After I went to school and began to learn, I think I slept longer.

I hardly remember any dreams during my teenage years, but I do remember a really intense dream when I was fifteen years old. I live in Jacksonville, Florida now and I know what tropical heat feels like. In the England I grew up in, the temperature never went above 75 fahrenheit (24 celsius), so I had no idea what real heat felt like. The first time I stepped off a plane, which was on the island of Ibiza in the Mediterranean, I was shocked by the wall of heat that hit me. I didn't even know the air could get that hot. What was interesting about this dream I had when I was fifteen, was that I was on a ship and the heat was like the heat you feel in Miami. In the dream I wasn't a fifteen year old boy, I was a man. We were sailing through a large river, with huge green trees all around us. The heat was humid and oppressive, although I had never felt tropical heat until I came to Florida, but the heat in the dream was exactly what you get in the Caribbean. We were watching and waiting for something, and I was aware of that in the dream. I was aware of other men on the ship with me, but that was all, nobody

134

was speaking. All of a sudden, another ship came at us, and men started boarding the ship. One man appeared next to me, and I just killed him. Bear in mind that I was a fifteen year old boy, and fifteen year old boys do not kill people. The interesting thing was that the person I was in the dream had no problems killing. He just did it. After he killed the first man, he killed two more. In the dream it was like being a passenger in another man's body. This man on the ship knew how to kill, and he was good at fighting. He felt no fear either. He went right into battle and he did what needed to be done. The colors in the dream were intense, and I awoke fairly quickly, but I was stunned by the way the person I had been in the dream had just killed other men without even thinking about it. There was no hesitation, he just did it.

When I was older I read a newspaper article about lucid dreaming, and I started to experiment and bought one or two books, and then I bought a few more books. Some books were useless, but some had information I could use. One thing that seemed to help encourage lucid dreams was to write down what you dreamed about immediately on waking up. I only did that once or twice, but I did concentrate on the dreams and think about them, and try to remember them. I found that once I did that, I could remember a dream I had been having on waking, and the next time I went to bed I could get back into that dream if I wanted. The same thing can happen if you go to the bathroom, you can jump right back into the dream you were having on waking, if you so desire.

There is also something called hypnagogic imagery, which is well documented by the medical profession. The word hypnagogic is based on the Greek word for sleep, and hypnagogic imagery refers to images that come as you drift into sleep. With practice, these images can become very clear and be in full color, and experimenting with this will also produce many more lucid dreams. In fact, I think this is the technique I first came across for producing dreams, and I became quite good at producing images after a few weeks of practice. I thought there would be a good Western site on hypnagogic imagery because it is a term recognized by the medical profession, but there is not. What I did find was that there is something called "yoga-nidra" (yogi sleep), which perfectly describes what I understand to be hypnagogic imagery. It goes further than just basic hypnagogic imagery, but the principle of keeping conscious awareness as you enter sleep appears to be the same. The link to this is here on Wikipedia. If you do not use Wikipedia, then try it because you can find just about anything on Wikipedia, and often you can find incredibly detailed and complex information in the articles. Here is the wiki link for yoga-nidra:

http://en.wikipedia.org/wiki/Yoga_Nidra

This describes the hypnagogic state pretty well. I am so used to it now that I can slip into something that can produce a dream fairly easily. If you are tired, as we all seem to be nowadays, then sleep will come and take you fairly quickly, but with practice you can keep some semblance of consciousness as the process of sleep kicks off. Having a target to visit such as a monastery or a mountain scene can be helpful. Abstract ideas work as well. I have tried things like going to visit the man who controls the world. This might sound weird, but it is a target to aim at, and it takes me somewhere in the dream state, and I can tell you that this man has pretty big palaces, whoever he is and wherever he lives. Trying this has produced some fairly intense dreams and like I said earlier, intense dreams are always relaxing.

Some of the books on out of body experiences have much better sections on how to produce lucid dreams than any of the books on lucid dreaming, and they are well worth trying. The best book I have ever read on lucid dreaming was written by a very down to earth young American called Sylvan Muldoon, who wrote the book back in the 1930s together with Hereward Carrington, who was a member of the British aristocracy. The book was called "The Projection of the Astral Body". Do not be put off by the title, for there is incredible information in this book that just cannot be found anywhere else, and many of the techniques for inducing lucid dreaming described by Sylvan Muldoon actually work. You can find this book on Amazon.

Once again if anyone has any questions or comments about lucid dreaming, I would love to hear from you, and I would like to hear about any experiences you have. My email address is at the end of the book and on my Amazon Author page.

Relaxation

I grew up in a Britain that does not exist anymore. When I grew up, most of the adults around me were relaxed most of the time. In the mid 1970s, quite a few people in California were working three day weeks, and still making a lot of money and we were told that soon everyone would be able to work three day weeks. Then we moved to the 1980s, where the mantra was to work as hard as the Japanese, and this has taken us to where we are now. It is never a good idea to try and push a foreign culture onto another country because often it does not produce the results expected. Something like one in two, or one in three, Americans is now on some kind of medication for stress. In Britain, it is one in ten people.

When I came to America my wife commented that I seemed to be able to relax much better than she could. Nowadays, after sixteen years in the United States, I'm not so sure. Everyone is encouraged to be busy, but I'm not sure how much actually gets done when people are stressed and tired. I have said before in this book, if governments do not look after the health of their people, then they face being controlled by other nations, and the West needs to be careful in this respect. Americans have never known a time when Europeans and Americans did not control the world, but six centuries ago, other nations came into Europe and pretty much did what they wanted.

Life in America, and Europe, needs to go back to a somewhat more carefree and relaxed life like we used to have. Perhaps we had this different life in those days because so many young men and women in the 1940s had their twenties controlled by World War II, that they made a conscious decision that their lives were going to be better. If the will of the people is strong enough in a certain direction, then what is important to them often overrules what the leaders of a country want to do, and often the people themselves know best.

There are things I used to do in England that I just don't do over here. I remember on beaches, just sitting on a rock and looking out over the water for hours. If you ever have a chance to do this, then try it, it is incredibly relaxing watching the waves hitting the shore. In England, I used to walk by rivers in the Derbyshire Peak District whenever I could. Some of the paths by rivers probably go back thousands of years because the easiest place to have a path is often next to a river. That is also why a lot of roads follow the course of a river. When we lived in Annapolis, Maryland my son, Nathan, and I would often drive up to the state parks around Frederick and Hagerstown. We would drive towards Hagerstown on Interstate 70, and as we neared Hagerstown we would see the West Maryland Mountains ahead of us. There is nothing like driving on a road, and seeing mountains ahead when you know you know you are going to be hiking in the area. Of the states I have lived in, or near, Maryland has the best state parks. I have never been out West, and I have heard that there are great state parks out there, but in the east around Washington D.C., the really good state parks are in Maryland, at least for me anyway. The ones we used to go to around the Frederick and Hagerstown area often had a lake in the middle, and we would usually hike and then end up with a walk around the lake. Up there I remember the walks were usually color coded and they told you the degree of difficulty, and all walks were usually fine for us, although we never hiked the Appalachian Trail, which I understand can be quite strenuous.

I remember in one park in Maryland, there were seven trails. The first six were all color coded, and the seventh was called the "Copperhead Trail". We were newly arrived in Maryland and had no idea what the word "copperhead" meant, but I had a good idea that it had nothing to do with mining. There are virtually no snakes in England, and there are no snakes in Alaska, so living in Annapolis was my first experience of living anywhere near snakes. I worked for an engineering company that was doing a huge multi-year engineering project at College Park just inside the beltway, and I used walk in the park area there at lunchtimes. One day I was talking to two young Indians, and I was telling them how a female student had just jogged past me, and disturbed a five foot long snake that came hurtling out of the bushes right in front of me, slid up a bridge, and dropped over the rail. It seemed more disturbed by me than I was of it, so I just kept still, and watched it while it went over the bridge. While we were talking one of the two Indians pointed to a tree with a large hole in the side about twenty feet up, and said that in India, they called trees like that snake trees because snakes lived in the holes in the tree. Just as we were looking at the tree, a six foot long snake slid out of the hole in the tree and went down the trunk. It was a long away so we just laughed and watched it go.

When my son Nathan was young I looked after him on my own, as I said earlier in the book, and one of the things I used to do was to make him laugh. I put a lot of effort into this because if you are a single parent, you have nobody to give you a break, and it made it a lot easier for me to be able to have him laugh. I found that there is a moment when you can stop a toddler crying by making him laugh, but you have to be alert and intervene before the real crying starts. I learnt to spiral him up into real heavy laughter, and even now we can be sitting in the main room, and we will hear roars of laughter coming from Nathan's room as he finds something funny on television. I think if you do that with your child it builds pathways in the brain, and the more the laughter pathways are stimulated, the more interconnections are built, and the happier your child can be when he or she grows up. I am a great believer that a lot of problems with teenagers are brought into existence by being too busy when the child is three years old, and ignoring them at an age when they are more easy to ignore.

I have wondered what kind of a world we could create, if for one just one generation, all the adults got together and decided they were all going to be nice to each other, so that nice behaviour was all the children ever saw. What would the children from a world like that be like I wonder? What would the world be like a hundred years later?

I think women will often do the right thing, but I think every society benefits if the men are self-sacrificing, and think of their families before they think of themselves. My father was like that, and my parents provided a safe, secure world for us at home so that we could go out from a solid home base. I have tried to do the same for my family, and I believe I have been successful in that. My step-daughter is the oldest, and I told her when she first moved out that she could come back anytime she wanted if things didn't work out, and that she could leave and return as often as she wanted. She did this a couple of times before renting her own place, and then getting married and setting up a secure home of her own, and I can tell by my granddaughter's face that she has a very secure and loving environment.

All the information for a man to learn how to be a good man exists in American society, and I am a better man for coming to America and living here. I am from another country and did not grow up here, and I don't think that information necessarily comes from the Church, I think it is just there in American society. If you look around the world, as I said before, women often do the right thing, and if the men are not prepared to raise the crops, then the women will always do it. There are some countries where the men are very industrious, and others where men spend their time sitting under trees. I cannot speak for women because I am a man, but if you are a man, it is important to create a safe, secure environment for your family. Do not go around looking for praise, just go ahead and do it and your family will appreciate it. If you are living on your own, then create a safe and secure environment, for yourself. There is a great book by a British man, James Allen, called "As a Man Thinketh", which was written in 1904. There are many versions of this book, but the best one is by James Allen and Marc Allen, and is called "As You Think". I mentioned Marc Allen earlier when I talked about using "quiet determination" as a way of making your way in the world. The phrase "quiet determination" is my phrase, but I believe it ties in with the philosophy Marc Allen uses. There is a lot of great wisdom in this book by James Allen and Marc Allen, both Eastern wisdom and Western wisdom, and I would strongly recommend you buy it.

The reason I talk about creating a safe and secure environment is because you will be healthier, and will fight type 2 diabetes far better, if everything around you is stable. My wife tells me from time to time that I brought stability into her life. Do not misunderstand what I say here because I think that she and her daughter had a fairly stable life before my son and I arrived, but perhaps I have brought something. My parents often used to run out of things, and when I was sixteen years old, I vowed that when I had my own house we would not run out of things, and it is very rare for that to happen. This is only a small thing, but you will have much more control over your life if you decide when you have to go to the store, rather than having to rush out at the last minute on a work evening when you don't really want to. A few years ago my step-daughter gave me a birthday card that said inside "Thank-you so much for all that you do". My wife was puzzled by this, and asked what our daughter meant by that. I said to her that there were things in the house that I just did, that nobody knew I did. She then challenged me by asking me to tell her one. In that situation my mind always goes blank, and I could only think of one thing. When I was a teenager, we would sit down to dinner together and the salt cellar would often be empty. Teenagers don't like getting up once they have sat down, so I decided at age fifteen that I would take over always filling the salt cellar so that it was never empty, and if it felt light to me while we were eating I would fill it at the end of the meal. When my wife put me on the spot by asking me to name something I did in the house that they didn't know about, all I could think of to say, was to ask her when she last filled a salt cellar. She looked blank for half a second, and then burst out laughing because the last time was probably a week or two before Nathan and I arrived in the country.

I do not believe that relaxation using alcohol, drugs, or legal drugs provided by the pharmaceutical companies is any help in long term relaxation. Relaxation must come from within. The Vikings in Scotland lived in a time when the climate was in a warm phase, and they were able to set their crops in the spring, and then go raiding all summer. Some of you will probably think the Vikings were barbarians, but theirs was a society where women were allowed to own land and had many rights that women do not even have in some countries right now, one thousand years later. There is a huge cathedral in South Wales called St. David's Cathedral, and my friend Dave and I once hiked down there. Like I said, Dave used to plan all the walks and I would make all the food, and I had never even heard of St. David's Cathedral. We stayed that weekend in Haverfordwest, which is where the actor Christian Bale grew up, and he was probably in his late teens and still living in Haverfordwest the weekend we were there. I thought I knew all the major towns in the UK but I had never heard of Haverfordwest, and it is actually quite a big town. We took a look round St. David's Cathedral, and Dave told me that it had been around in Viking times, and that the Vikings had raided it so much that the cathedral was moved inland. We took a walk near the coast, which was quite rocky, but there was one small beach in a tiny inlet, and I realized that must have been where the Vikings landed because it was the only area for a considerable distance where you could land Viking longboats. It was an interesting feeling to stand on a beach where Vikings had once stood, and to think about it. It is very unlikely that any Viking who landed there would have been an ancestor of mine, but some of my ancestors very probably spoke the same language as the Vikings that stood on the beach one thousand years ago. On the Orkney Islands and the Shetland Islands in the north of Scotland, the people spoke a language called "Norn" until the eighteenth century, which is closely related to Norwegian.

I guess where I am going with this is to say that if you want to really relax, you have to get out of the city. In my opinion, mankind would be better off without cities. They are an aberration in our history, and the freedoms of men and women who live in cities are certainly much less than the freedoms enjoyed by nomads. You may say, well how do nomads find enough food, but that is only because cities have taken the land that once belonged to nomads. There has been much speculation as to why mankind took 100,000 years to have civilization, but the answer to that question is almost certainly hostile climate. Every planet and moon in the solar system with an atmosphere has winds, but our planet, at the moment, has some of the lowest wind speeds in the solar system. On Neptune, the winds were measured by Voyager 2 in 1989 at 1,300 miles an hour, and tiny little Mars can whip up a dust storm that can cover the whole planet in a matter of days, even though it has quite a thin atmosphere. Many of the planets and large moons have winds in the hundreds of miles an hour, and some of them have winds approaching 1,000 miles an hour. There is probably no way in paleontology to measure wind speeds, except to look at a destructive event, and guess, but even then it would be hard, so we just don't know what wind speeds have been like in the past. I have noticed that the winds in the high atmosphere above Jacksonville have been moving much faster than they used to when we first came here. This change occurred in August 2011, and has not yet gone away. Perhaps it is a momentary aberration in the life of the planet, or a harbinger of things to come. My son and I take the dog for a walk every night, and we often watch clouds racing across the sky at what are, for this latitude, quite considerable speeds. Perhaps I am wrong, and the winds have always been like this above Jacksonville, but they certainly were not like that when we first came here.

There seems to be a movement afoot in the world to get the last remaining nomads off their land, and into towns and cities, but I think that would be a bad thing, and I also think that mankind as a whole would lose a lot if we lost some of those old traditions. Also, if there ever comes a time when all our crops fail, then we, in the cities, will need the nomads to show us how to survive. Nothing empties a city faster than a ten year famine, and if you don't think that could happen to us, then be aware that just about every civilization in the last six thousand years never thought it could crash, but most of them are gone. The last six hundred years have seen vast flows of wealth out of the rest of the world and into Europe, but recently all the wealth has started to flow the other way, and Europe now faces a tipping point in its near future. That tipping point will not be pretty, and is likely to be a time of fast and sudden change, and possibly mass starvation even though that may be unthinkable now. Europe is currently about to see this time of massive change at a time when some of our politicians in the West are just shadows of the men who have governed Europe in the past. Sometime in the next twenty years, men and women in Britain may well ask, where is Winston Churchill now when we need him the most, for there is no doubt that during World War II Britain was lucky to have Winston Churchill. It is often forgotten in Britain that Winston Churchill had an American mother, and I do not know as much about him as I should, but he was certainly a man of grand visions who was capable of dreaming lofty dreams for his country.

We have created a civilization where it is hard for people to be different, and hard for people not to be sucked into what used to be called the rat race. Much study has been done cramming rats into smaller and smaller spaces, and when you do that, chaos and violence rises in the rat population. There is actually a lot of land on this planet, and before the concept of land ownership arose, I believe everybody had plenty of land. Now, many of us are crammed into small spaces, and that leads to stress and pressure. You may have no choice but to live in a city or a densely packed suburb, but you should do your best to get out of the city, or suburb, at least once a month. America's state parks are incredible places, and are available to any American citizen for a very small fee. Avail yourself of them, for a day spent in a good state park is a day in a completely different world than a day in front of the television. If you are hiking, then your phone should always be switched off, and the real world should not be allowed to intrude. In fact, a better definition would more likely be that when you are in a state park, you are in the real world, and when you are in a city, you are not in the real world at all. Cities may be full of glamour and glitz, but at the end of the day they can leave you feeling empty inside. I have often driven through the English countryside early in the morning. There are often farms beside the road, and if you are out early enough, some of the farm animals are up and others are still lying asleep, and it is interesting to see that. There are many young people in cities who have never seen a farm animal. That used to be a big thing in England when I was young, I don't know whether it is in America. One of the best days I ever had as a child was going to a farm with my cousins, and sliding down the hay bales that the farmer had stacked in the barn. I must have been young because I still had shorts on, and even though the hay made scratches on my legs I still kept sliding. It is important to seek pleasure outdoors because we are made to be outdoors, and sitting behind glass all day is probably not healthy.

There is an American called Jon Turk. I have three of his books, and the first one I bought was called "The Raven's Gift: A Scientist, a Shaman, and Their Remarkable Journey Through the Siberian Wilderness". This is an incredible book, and well worth buying. Sometimes people think that they can't afford books, but if you take your wife out to dinner in America it will typically cost $30 to $40, and sometimes a lot more. The next day the meal is gone and there is nothing to show for it, but if you spend the money on a book then you will have something to show for it. If you think you can't afford books but you go out to eat ten times a month, which is pretty normal in the United States, then divert one or two of those meals towards book purchases. Jon Turk was a scientist with a Ph.D. in organic chemistry. He was spending his life underground studying particles when he decided he wanted his freedom. As I said earlier, this world we live in discriminates against anyone who wants their freedom, and that discrimination is as harsh as you will find anywhere in society.

You may as well be a leper as decide you don't want to have a normal job. Jon Turk was lucky enough to have his freedom. He did this by writing scientific textbooks, and when money was short, by working fishing boats in Alaska and the like. The rest of his life he spent exploring, in an age where exploring is discouraged by individuals working on their own. That life at times has been a hard life, in one section he describes talking to his doctor before a lone kayaking trip in a remote part of the world, to find out how to put his shoulder joint back into place if he pulled it out, as there would be nobody to do it for him. If I remember correctly, he did have to do that at one point on the journey. "The Raven's Gift: A Scientist, a Shaman, and Their Remarkable Journey Through the Siberian Wilderness" is an incredible book and describes a trip to a Siberian shaman on the Kamchatka Peninsula in Russia. I am not going to go into details about the book, I will leave that to you, but it is a fascinating read. One of the interesting things in the book is that the word for raven in the native Siberian language is almost exactly the same as the word for raven in the language the Native Alaskans use. It would be, of course, because the Native Americans came from Siberia, but it is interesting to see words like that in the language.

It is important that we treasure the open areas and the state parks that we do have left. I believe that the reason America has left Alaska virtually untouched, by comparison with the lower 48, is because the country realizes just how fast the white man overran what had been kept pristine by the Native Americans. The Native American rule was to take only what you need and leave the rest untouched, which is a philosophy that has never existed in many places in the rest of the world. Our world gets smaller every day, and we are many, far too many now. When Chief Seattle made his address to the white people who had come to take his land, he supposedly said that they should be careful with the land lest they ruin it. A Scotsman, John Muir, in despair about the way forestry companies were trashing the land of the American People, once plucked up his courage, walked up to President Theodore Roosevelt's hotel bedroom door in the middle of the night, and slid a letter underneath asking the President to intervene. The result was the introduction of state parks.

When I first came to America not many Americans had heard of the British television show Doctor Who. Many more Americans have seen it now, and quite a few of my son's friends watch it. I remember one show that made a lasting impression on me. Star Trek had a kind and benevolent Federation, except on one memorable episode when Spock had a beard and was actually quite scary, but on Doctor Who they often had the "Terran Empire", which tended to enslave planets. On one show the Doctor's ship, the Tardis, was in orbit around a subjugated planet. The planet had been industrialized, and thick, heavy, dark gray smog hung over the whole planet. One of the Doctor's assistants commented that the planet looked disgusting from space, and the doctor told her that if she thought that looked bad, then she should see Earth. It is very much up to us to make sure nobody can ever say that about our planet. There are wonderful places out in nature that can inspire incredible thoughts in us. Much is said about terraforming planets to make them inhabitable for mankind, but we are on a very bad path, and if we are not careful, then the first planet we will have to terraform for mankind to live on could well be our own.

I have a lot of great memories, and I treasure those memories. Many of the best days of my life have been spent outside. When it is time to move onto the next world, then your memories should not be of the television programs you have watched, or the expensive meals you have eaten, they should be of the outdoors. Remember that, and it will serve you well in your quest for relaxation.

Meditation

I think there is a lot more to meditation than we are told when we study transcendental meditation. There is a book out there called "The Yoga Sūtras of Patañjali". The title means the yoga threads of Patanjali, and "sūtras" is the same root word that we derive the word "sutures" from in America for surgical stitches. There are many different versions of "The Yoga Sūtras of Patañjali". I have a friend who spent six weeks in India studying under B.K.S Iyengar, and he told me the best one to get was the one by Swami Satchidananda who runs Yogaville in Virginia. The Yoga Sūtras of Patañjali is an interesting book. In the book, Patanjali refers to "Siddhis", or powers, that come to those who meditate and practice a lot. The book then states that the Siddhis should be ignored, and that they are a distraction. I am just one man, but I do not believe this is correct. What if they are wrong, and one of our purposes on this planet is to seek the Siddhis, or powers, and use them. I have heard that people who meditate for hours at a time sometimes have really strange experiences, but I do not know anyone who has done this.

It is a while since I have read The Yoga Sūtras of Patañjali. If I remember correctly, the references to the Siddhis are almost magical, but at the end of the day there is no guide for actually getting from A to B. Having said that, I have always wanted to spend six hours in one day meditating, but given the state of our busy society this is not necessarily a practical thing to do unless you are young, and a student and have more time.

I will say one thing; the Western books I have read tend to give you actual information about how to do things that you can apply for yourself. Many of the books on dowsing (or water divining) were written by senior officers in the British military during the days of the British Empire, for the simple reason that many of the areas that the British took control of were in desert regions, or regions with low water. Finding a water source, and digging a well for 500 troops under your command could be the difference between life and death. In the days of the Russian Empire, the Russians often rode hundreds of miles to attack in very bad conditions. In one of the earliest Russian expeditions into what is now Kazakhstan, the Russians used hundreds of camels to take an army and supplies across the desert. They used camels because horses could not have crossed the land they planned to cross. It was spring and the winter should have been over, but there was a late season snowstorm and many of the camels froze to death. Most of the army was butchered by the people they had come to conquer. It was almost 100 years before the Russians tried again, but the next time they were successful, and the result of that was a march across Asia, the likes of which had never been seen before and may never be seen again. When Russian expansion slowed down they had reached the Pacific Ocean, although they even crossed that, and many places in Alaska have Russian names because it was once part of the Russian Empire. When I lived in Alaska, I worked with some Alaska natives who were descended partly from Russians and there are Russian Orthodox churches all over Alaska.

I mentioned above that many of the books on dowsing were written by British army officers, and archaeologist Tom Lethbridge learnt how to dowse from a book written by a British army officer. It is almost certain that Lethbridge's interest in dowsing arose because he was an archaeologist, and he may well have used it in his profession, although we will never know that because to write about it would have the kiss of death for his career. All Lethbridge's books about dowsing were written after he retired and his pension was secure. The reason I have said this, is because often books from certain areas of the East lack practical instructions on how to do something. There is always plenty of talk about miraculous things, but never the simple set of instructions that say if you do this, this, and this, then the following will happen.

In one of Lethbridge's books, he talked about an archaeological trip to Greenland. The Viking settlements on Greenland are the only European colony which completely failed, and they were destroyed by the climate during the mini ice age in mediaeval times. Vikings lived in Greenland alongside Eskimos, in fact, I recently read that Eskimos used to visit and land on the northwest part of Scotland in an area called Cape Wrath (it is called Cape Wrath for very good reasons). It is possible that if the mini ice age had become worse, that Scotland would now have Eskimos living there. In case anyone is thinking the term should be Inuit, not Eskimo, then I worked with Eskimos in Alaska, and that was the name they used to refer to themselves. Besides which, most Inuit live in Canada, and the people I worked with were Yupiks, and Iñupiats, and I don't even know whether there are any Inuit in Alaska. The Yupiks live in Siberia in Russia, and in western and South-central Alaska. The Iñupiats live on, or near, the North Slope (northern coastal area) in Alaska, and also in the interior of Alaska.

The Vikings and the Eskimos in Greenland did not really understand each other. The Vikings referred to the Eskimos as "skraelings", which means wretches in English, and the Eskimos thought that the Vikings were descended from Eskimo women who had mated with dogs because they were so hairy. We will never know if any of the Vikings were taken in by the Eskimos, unless we can find their DNA in the population of Greenland. When Lethbridge was in Greenland it was the 1930s, and it was a very different place then than now. Lethbridge was fascinated by native cultures, and felt we could learn a lot from them and that is true, one of the main reasons Roald Amundsen beat Robert Falcon Scott to the South Pole was because he had noticed that Eskimos with dog teams could move much faster on the ice than white men with horses.

Lethbridge told a story in the book about a British party that shot a polar bear to eat while they were on the ice. A group of Eskimo hunters stopped to talk to them, and told the British party that the polar bear was good to eat but warned them not to eat the liver under any circumstances. Of course, the British ignored the Eskimos, and ate the whole polar bear. Polar bears eat seals, which eat fish, and as a result the polar bear ingests huge amounts of vitamin A from the seals it eats. All that vitamin A gets stored in the polar bear's liver, and is actually at toxic levels. Lethbridge mentioned that after the British party ate the polar bear's liver they retired to their tents, and all of them fell into comas and did not wake up until two or three days later.

One of the other interesting things Lethbridge mentioned, was that when he was in Greenland he was one of three archaeologists, and one of the British men was 6 feet 6 inches tall. The local Eskimo chief came out to talk to them, selected the tall British archaeologist, and asked him if he would sleep with his daughter. The reason for this goes back to our limited human DNA, and all the problems it causes. The Eskimos were well aware of this issue, and were always looking for people from outside groups to introduce DNA into the local tribes. I once shared an office on the North Slope at Kuparuk in Alaska with an Eskimo woman in her twenties called Violet, and I asked her about this and she said it was true. Then she told me she had Brazilian blood because one of her ancestors had a child with a Brazilian sailor, who was in a ship that had stopped at Point Hope in Alaska where she was from. It was really interesting sharing an office with her, it is always interesting to hear about other cultures. The Eskimos are known for their intelligence, and they run a lot of companies in the oilfields of Alaska. In fact, Houston Contracting, the company I worked for was owned by an Eskimo holding company from Barrow in Alaska, and one of the Vice Presidents at Houston told me that the Eskimos were very intelligent and were good businessmen, which shows what can happen when native groups are given a chance in the United States. If anyone reads this book from Point Hope in Alaska, or knows Violet from Point Hope then please give her my email address from the back of the book because I would love to hear from her and hear how she is doing. We worked together for a month or two, and then she went home for the Point Hope annual whale hunt and I lost touch with her.

One in every five or every six people in Alaska was an Alaska Native (Athabaskan Indians and Eskimos). The Athabaskan language runs through the Alaska interior, and through Canada, and is closely related to the language spoken by the Apaches in the southern United States. I remember one time I pulled up in the parking lot of the Anchorage Barnes and Noble, and there were a couple of Alaska Natives who were a little under the influence of alcohol. The people that pulled up near me rushed into the store as fast as possible. From my experience in England, I can tell the difference between a happy drunk and one who might turn dangerous and want to fight, and the two Alaska Natives were definitely in the former category. One of them said hello to me as I walked past and I stopped to talk to them. We talked for over half an hour, and they had a really good sense of humor and we shared quite a few jokes.

Alaska was a really interesting place to live. There was a cinema there on Fireweed Avenue, with a huge screen that could hold 1,500 people at a time, and I have been there when it has been full. I also saw more foreign films in Alaska than I have seen anywhere else in the United States. All the cinemas in Jacksonville get together and decide what to show, and they all tend to show (or block) the same films, which restricts choice whereas in Alaska they went for diversity. There was one bear for every ten people in Alaska, and I remember once flying in from the North Slope and going out to Hatcher Pass with my wife. I wanted to go for a walk and we started out, but then she told me that the bears could be coming out of hibernation and would be hungry, and she wanted to go back to the car. I walked her back to the restaurant where we had parked and then when she went into the restaurant, I went back out onto the trail. However, the whole point of hiking is to relax, and when your wife has just told you that if you meet a black bear on the trail, it will turn you into lunch, then it is difficult to relax. I don't carry a gun and I didn't even have a knife, and some of the black bears in Alaska are five feet tall on two legs, and weigh upwards of 330 pounds. I walked about a mile before I turned back. If I had been carrying a good sharp long knife such as a Scottish dirk, which is as long as a man's forearm then I might have carried on, but the idea of being attacked and not even being able to fight back bothered me. If you die, you die, but if that happens then you should at least take whatever attacked you on to the next world with you.

The title of this section was meditation. I think meditation can be useful, but I do think some of the claims for it may be a little overblown. A claim that violence in an area goes down if 1% of the population meditates is interesting, but I would like to hear an American police officer's viewpoint on that if it was carried out in his area. Of all the things I have learnt over the years involved with stimulating different areas of the mind, meditation may be the one I have used the least.

I once experimented with clairvoyance after reading a book by a British writer, W.E. Butler. I lacked the money for expensive paraphernalia like a crystal, or a crystal ball, both of which are expensive (I was in my mid twenties), and I used a sheet of white photocopy paper instead. If you look at a sheet of white paper for ten to twenty minutes every morning, or every evening, then after about one month faces and images will appear on the paper. My first wife hated me trying anything like that so I think I stopped after a while, but it did create certain additional pathways in my brain. Shortly after that, I parked in the parking lot in Burton-on-Trent town center where we lived. Parking was tight there, and you actually had to pay until 8 pm. It was 7:40 pm, and a complete waste of money to buy a parking ticket so I didn't bother as I was only going to be in the store for ten minutes. As I was walking across the parking lot, I heard a voice in my head, which was from my subconscious that said "I wonder if you will get a parking ticket". I ignored it, as you would, and when I came out ten minutes later, there was a notice on my car windshield specifying the fine I would be about to pay. I did not ignore that voice again, and let me be clear, this is not a voice, it is more like a thought in my head. As I have said before in this book, if you practice dowsing, or tarot reading, or clairvoyance, or any of the other multitudes of different experiments I have done over the years, then the barrier between the subconscious mind and the conscious mind breaks down, and this is to your advantage. Let me explain this in the next paragraph, American women that my wife and I have told this next story to really like this story because it is something that can happen to anybody.

In 1996, my son Nathan and I went to the English Lake District for the first time, with a friend called Geoff and his family. I loved the area, but felt we spent too much time in the hotel and not enough outdoors. My mother had an operation shortly after that, and when she was able to get about again, I said I would take her for a weekend away. I took her, Nathan, and my Hungarian au-pair Erika, up to the Lake District. My mother, Nathan, and Erika went to the hotel lounge while I unpacked my things and Nathan's things (he was six at the time). As I was unpacking, my hotel room door was open, and I heard a foreign woman (an American – this was my future wife Cecilia) trying to book into the hotel. The manager was saying that they were fully booked, and that there would be no rooms available for at least two weeks. They carried on talking and I carried on unpacking. I left the room a few minutes later, and I was heading to the lounge at the other end of the hotel to join my mother, Nathan, and Erika. As I was walking across the foyer I got the same "voice" (or thought) in my head from my subconscious, that I told you about earlier. The voice basically said "you should go and talk to her". Once again this is not a real voice, just a thought that comes from my subconscious. By then I knew that listening to these messages from my subconscious were always to my advantage. The American woman was standing on her own in the hotel lobby looking at the brochures. I changed direction in mid stride and walked towards her. I had no idea what I was going to say, so I just walked up and said that they had pretty good brochures in the hotel. She agreed with me, and then we got to talking. She took me outside to meet her friend Irene who she was travelling with. I had never really talked to American women before, and I was stunned by how charming and nice they both were. We talked for about forty minutes before they had to go, but before they left I told them I had enjoyed talking and that we should exchange addresses. They both gave me their addresses and phone numbers, and I said I would write to them. Before she left the UK Cecilia called me and we chatted for about an hour, and then when she went back to Alaska we talked on the phone. She is a teacher, and had originally been in the UK for a teacher exchange with a teacher from England called Jean. We talked during the fall, and Cecilia said she was planning to come over and visit Jean at Christmas, and she would come up and see me while she was over. The trip to Jean fell through, and she asked if she could stay with Nathan and I in Nottingham. She came over for three weeks at Christmas, and I ended up flying to Alaska three weeks after that and we were married. There is a picture of us at the Lake Lucille Inn where we had the reception, where we are standing next to a stuffed grizzly bear that they had in the foyer. I am one inch under six feet tall, and the bear's outstretched arms come to just above my head so you can imagine how big the bears in Alaska are. I would like to pay tribute to Cecilia here for giving me so many happy years. We have been married for sixteen years now. I always said that anyone who married as fast as that was a fool, but it is the best thing I ever did. However, if I had ignored the voice from my subconscious, we would never have even talked let alone gotten married.

Last Comments

After this section you will find Appendix 1, which is a follow on from the chapter "Climbing out of Diabetes". Appendix 1 covers my climb out of diabetes in much more detail with all my blood sugar numbers listed. Although this may take some working through, it is something that can help motivate you and also help at the times you are pushing hard against the tipping points because you can see setbacks in my numbers and then my victory. This came fairly quickly, and one thing you will also see is the effect of going on vacation to Aruba part way through the fight. Over there I had no control over what I ate apart from the obvious like avoiding things with sugar in. My blood sugar pushed higher again as a result of that, but that is good information because it shows you what can happen if you drop your guard, or you are in a position where circumstances give you less control over your situation.

In Aruba I was unable to exercise like I had done, although I did manage to walk. When you take your blood sugar numbers keep all of them, even the bad ones because a bad number can often tell you a lot. I have said elsewhere that my blood sugar number was almost always higher on a Monday morning than on a Tuesday morning, and that really tells you that taking less exercise, and eating in restaurants will give you a higher number. I wish I had kept more of a note of what I was eating, but I always found it difficult to write down everything I ate, whereas writing down how many weights I lifted, or how many stairs I climbed, was much easier for some reason.

Do not underestimate the effect that walking long distances will have on your blood sugar. Some of the largest muscles in the body are in the legs, and consequently they burn a lot of blood sugar when they are used extensively. I think the key to this is that the body can always manage thirty to forty minutes of exercise quite easily, but once you go over that period you start to drain the blood sugar reservoirs in the body. Once again, if you have never exercised do not go out and walk five miles, start slowly and build up. I know a young woman who was probably thirty at the most, who went to a theme park and walked seven miles around the park, which is the distance round the circuit. The next day one of her legs was swollen. She was not overweight and that probably happened because she never exercised. She was young, and if you are older, you have to be careful. Having said that, you are descended from generations of men and women who routinely walked ten to twenty miles a day, so it is in your genetic heritage to be able to do that, and you can bring it back by building up slowly. I am not suggesting you walk those kinds of distances, you should not need to, but it does need to be stated that you are perfectly capable of walking that far. There were five children in my mother's family, and when she was young in the 1930s they would often walk to the opposite side of town to see relatives, which must have been at least seven or eight miles. Although there were buses, my grandparents probably saw no need to spend money on seven bus tickets when it could have been better spent on food or clothes, as the 1930s was a decade of austerity.

Although I don't know how many people this book can help, it will really give me a lot of pleasure if this book pulls a significant percentage of you out of type 2 diabetes. I believe that we are all put on this Earth to help each other. The procedures in this book are not rocket science, and they are all natural things we used to do until we developed "civilization", and began to live in towns and cities. Although there is great benefit to things such as parks and libraries, not everything civilization brings is beneficial, and type 2 diabetes is a prime example of that. Somewhere, there is a tipping point that remains unseen, and something we have done in the last thirty years has triggered that tipping point because when I was growing up, type 2 diabetes was almost unknown except among the elderly, and when I say elderly I mean people seventy or older. My grandmother was probably at least seventy-five when she developed type 2 diabetes, and she may have been older than that. If she were around now, I wonder if diabetes would come much earlier, perhaps in her forties and we need to research exactly why that is happening. Some people assume that it is only overweight people that get type 2 diabetes, but that is not true, it is striking plenty of thin people and in some ways it hits them harder because many thin people are not used to exercising, whereas people who have had to fight weight gain often have experience of exercising.

I would like to call for further research from universities around the world, and I would like to ask those universities to make routine checks of people who do not have type 2 diabetes, so that we can build up a really good database of blood sugar levels in the general population. A good experiment would be to take one hundred men and one hundred women, and have them take their morning blood sugars for a month. We could do this at ages twenty, twenty-five, thirty, thirty-five and so on every five years. We have no idea what happens to a twenty year old jock after a night of heavy drinking and partying. Is his blood sugar normal, or is it higher the next morning even though he does not have diabetes? Those are questions we should know the answers to, but we probably don't. We can theorize that since the jock is fit and healthy, then his numbers would be normal, but what if they are higher on the day after the party than all the other days of the week? What if his normal blood sugar in the morning is 83 mg/dl (4.31 mmol/L), but on that day, it is 87 mg/dl (4.83 mmol/L)? We need to know things like that because patterns can be built up, and to use my jigsaw analogy, pieces can be put onto the board and interconnections can be made.

What about comparing the blood sugars of young university students in America with young university students in Saudi Arabia, where young people do not drink alcohol. Would that make a difference? Is there a difference between Swedes and Norwegians, even though they are all Scandinavians? We need to build up databases that tell us these things, and then maybe, just maybe, somewhere in one of those databases, will be the tipping point that is causing this outbreak of diabetes. I am an expert at finding anomalies in data, I am an accountant and I have spent my whole career doing that. If there is one number that is different in one hundred numbers, then I can usually find it very quickly.

At the moment we seem to be just blindly accepting that type 2 diabetes is on the increase, but something massive must have changed to do that. Is it happening in every country or just some countries? These are things we should already be looking at because the costs of type 2 diabetes are going to cripple some of our economies in the next thirty years. That's not my problem, but it is my government's problem. If 50% of all the adults over fifty develop diabetes, how do we compete effectively with other countries?

Appendix 2 has a link to a converter that converts United States blood sugar numbers to United Kingdom blood sugar numbers, and I have also listed the equivalent UK numbers to 80 mg/dl and 126 mg/dl. Most of continental Europe uses the same scale as the United States and measures in mg/dl. The UK uses mmol/L (millimoles per liter). If you are a UK reader of this book, I would use at least two decimal places when you put your blood sugar levels onto a spreadsheet, as you need to see small incremental changes. For example a blood sugar level of 81 mg/dl is equivalent to 4.50 mmol/L and a blood sugar level of 82 mg/dl is equivalent to 4.56 mmol/L.

Appendix 3 has a link to a healing technique called the Dynamind Technique. This has been developed by Serge Kahili King from Hawaii. To quote Serge's own words:

"The Dynamind Technique is based on a theory that all physical, emotional and mental problems are related to excessive tension in the body. The theory proposes that tension accumulates in layers, with focal points that produce specific symptoms. Healing takes place when tension layers are relaxed."

In my opinion, this is well worth trying. It takes just a few minutes and costs you nothing, so give it a try. I said elsewhere in this book that when I began to investigate the things in the world that science chose to ignore, I found a mixture of things that worked and things that did not. Everything I have tried from Serge King's books has worked, and some of those things that have worked cannot be explained by Western science. I don't know Serge King and I have never met him, but I am a great believer that if something works then that knowledge should be passed on.

This has been an interesting book to write, and enjoyable to research. I especially enjoyed researching the part about glucose transporters. I had read about Glucose Transporter 4 several years ago, but at the time I only had two articles and there is so much more information out there now. I mentioned in the chapter about relaxation and dreaming that when I was young I would go out in my dreams to help people, and that has always been part of my philosophy of life. Like I said above, I believe that we are all put on this planet to help each other and make the world better. Perhaps I am a little naïve, but I believe that the world was meant to be filled with parks and libraries, and that somewhere mankind has gotten off track.

I would love to hear from you about whether this book helps you fight off type 2 diabetes. Please email me at the email address at the end of the book, and tell me about your experiences. I would far rather be reading a letter from you than reading the news, which tends to be almost the same every day. At work I get a real kick out of improving things or cutting the time someone has to spend doing a job, and in the same way I hope that this book will help you.

Good luck, and may your God go with you.

Michael Ward
Jacksonville, Florida
March 2013

Email address:

jfi_mward@hotmail.com

(There is an underscore after the jfi in my email address)

Amazon's Michael Ward Page http://www.amazon.com/-/e/B007A550QM

Website: www.sites.google.com/site/michaelwardwriter

Follow me on Twitter at: https://twitter.com/Michael56984009

Books by Michael Ward

Non-Fiction

Type 2 Diabetes: How to Kick its Ass

Novels

The Banker With a Face Full of Evil – Scandinavian Crime Novel

Short Story Books

SHORTS - Five Free Short Stories
SHORTS 2 - Five Short Stories
SHORTS 3 - Five Free Short Stories
SHORTS 4 - Five Free Short Stories

Lisa Molin Assassin Series

Lisa Molin Assassin – One Hell of an Execution in Tallinn in Estonia
Lisa Molin Assassin – One Hell of an Execution in the Frisian Islands
Lisa Molin Assassin – The Execution of a Spaniard in Ibiza
Lisa Molin Assassin – The Execution of a Man From Stuttgart in Hawaii
Lisa Molin Assassin – The Night Train from Switzerland
Lisa Molin Assassin – The Execution of a Vice President in Sweden
Lisa Molin Assassin – The Execution of a Drug Dealer Dressed as Saddam
Lisa Molin – A Hit Ordered by a Woman from London
Lisa Molin – A Quiet Kill in Interlaken

Dangerous Scotsman Series

A Dangerous Scotsman in Afghanistan
A Dangerous Scotsman in Tajikistan

Jacksonville Jack Series (writing as Peter Brennan)

Jacksonville Jack
Jacksonville Jack – Moonrise
Jacksonville Jack – Helen in Georgia

Assassin Stephen Haggerty Series

Assassination in Washington D.C.
Assassination in Miami
Assassination in Anchorage, Alaska – due out 2013

Individual Short Stories

The Conquest of France AD 2013
The Vampire Who Sold Houses
The Civilization of the Ravens
Judgment Day is Today and it Begins in Miami
The House That Collected Realtors
Blowback
England is the Property of New Delhi
Your Mission is to Kill Saint Paul on Malta
Siberian Shamans
The Beach at the End of Time
Sharing a Life With a Kindred Spirit
My Name is Pawan (The Wind) and Soon all of you Will Know
my Name
Summoning the Wrath of God
The Devil Came Down to Georgia
Storming the compound of a Rich Man – an American Revolution
Story
Chinese Armageddon
City of the New South
An Artist in this Life

Michael Ward's books are published by Amazon and Barnes and Noble

Website: www.sites.google.com/site/michaelwardwriter

Amazon's Michael Ward Page http://www.amazon.com/-/e/B007A550QM

Barnes and Noble Nook – there is no author page – search for books by typing the name of the book in http://www.barnesandnoble.com/u/nook/379003208

Blood Sugar Numbers and Exercise Numbers for Climbing out of Diabetes

In this appendix I am going to document my blood sugar numbers in detail for the period when I attacked and vanquished type 2 diabetes. As I have said throughout this book, type 2 diabetes is your enemy and you must adopt that kind of thinking when you go into the attack. If you suffer setbacks, then you go in harder. Persistence is the key here, and the aim is to drain your blood sugar reserves. I decided to publish all the blood sugar numbers I had taken just so that you can see that there were good days and bad days, and good numbers and bad numbers. In the end, persistence won through and my numbers just flipped into normal levels.

I will go through week by week and analyze what happened in that week. I found that my morning blood sugar readings were the last to move into the normal range. I have records giving the date and time of day of each reading and I will list the times because that may be useful to you. Days of the week will also be listed just for the reason that I exercised five days a week and tended to relax at the weekends both with exercise and food. However, with food I still used some common sense. If you put in a lot of hard work in the week, and then have a big bowl of ice cream at the weekend, then you have just taken five steps back for the seven steps you have just taken forward.

I went back into my exercise spreadsheet, and I now see that it starts on Thanksgiving Day, which was 22 November, 2007. I didn't start taking my blood sugar until a week or two after starting exercising and the first blood sugar reading I have is on Saturday December 8, 2007. I started the weeks on a Monday and ran them through until midnight on Sunday nights. A much briefer version of this is in the chapter called "Climbing out of Diabetes" but I felt there would be some readers who would like to see everything in detail so here it is.

Week Ending Sunday November 25, 2007

All I have for this week is exercise records. This was the week of Thanksgiving and after Thanksgiving Day we went to Disney for a few days. I must have still been determined to exercise because over the four days I walked 14.8 miles, I climbed 10 flights of stairs, and I lifted a few weights on Thanksgiving Day but nothing much. I would like to see every hotel with a good set of weights in its exercise room, and two weight benches so that two people could work out so if you are reading this, and you work for a hotel chain please put the idea forward to management.

Week Ending Sunday December 2, 2007

Again, all I have for this week are exercise records, but now I started to get into it. I walked 16.5 miles this week, and I walked five days out of the week. I climbed 20 flights of stairs. I even went down with a tape measure and measured the height of the stairs I was climbing. This came out at 14 feet, so my estimated height climbed was 280 feet. I didn't lift any weights that week, or if I did, I didn't record it.

Week Ending Sunday December 9, 2007

This week I have exercise records and a few blood sugar records too. I was sick the first three days of the week with the flu so I ramped the exercise up towards the end of the week. I walked 16.0 miles and climbed 20 flights of stairs. This was the first week I really started lifting weights, and I did 750 forward wrist curls, 450 reverse wrist curls, 320 concentration curls, 130 single arm extensions, and 60 side bends. These were all done on each side so that means I did 750 forward wrist curls on my right arm, and another 750 on my left arm. This sounds a lot, but you really can do those fairly quickly. I do one arm at a time because I like to concentrate fully on making sure I have the right form, and it is easier to do that if you work one arm at a time. I do 10 reps on each arm, and as I work one arm the other arm is resting, and then I can go back and work it again straight away. This is not necessarily the right way to build muscle, but it is the right way to burn blood sugar. If you are unfamiliar with weight lifting then concentration curls work the biceps, and single arm extensions work the triceps.

My blood sugar records for the week are as follows. Readers in areas other than the United States should note that in the US, the month comes first in the date, and then the day of the month:

Saturday 12-08-07, 3:27pm 120 mg/dl (6.67 mmol/L), 6:59pm 108 mg/dl (6.0 mmol/L)

These results for Saturday are interesting. They are done after exercising, and not in the morning, but they are both technically under the blood sugar range limit of 126 mg/dl, although the one at 3:27pm is only just under. Bear in mind that just over a month earlier in October 2007, I had three numbers all in the 200 range on the week that I found that I had type 2 diabetes. That week when my step-daughter took my blood sugar the number was 255 mg/dl (14.17 mmol/L). An hour later, after walking 1.9 miles it was only 10 points lower at 245 mg/dl (13.61 mmol/L), and then a few days later when I had the morning blood test, it was 293 mg/dl (16.28 mmol/L). The morning blood sugar was 40 to 50 mg/dl higher. I wish I had taken my blood sugar during November, but I have said elsewhere that I probably just did not want to see a number anywhere near 293 mg/dl. This is a pity because it would have been useful to have some higher numbers, and then see the progression downwards. Let's look at Sunday's blood sugar numbers next.

Sunday 12-08-07, 11:30am 126 mg/dl (7.0 mmol/L), 12:16pm 136 mg/dl (7.56 mmol/L), 5:36pm 115 mg/dl (6.39 mmol/L), 10:08pm 134 mg/dl (7.44 mmol/L)

This is interesting too because only one of these numbers is in range. I could technically say that the first one was in range at 126 mg/dl but I'm going to call that one out of range because it is right on the limit. At the top I listed the total for the week for exercise. Now I'm going to go in and look at Saturday and Sunday individually. As I said earlier, I was sick for three days at the start of the week. On Thursday, I walked 2.4 miles, which was the first walking I did that week. On Saturday I walked 8.0 miles. I don't normally walk that distance, but there is no doubt I was playing catch up for not having done anything that week. I said in the conclusion not to underestimate the effect of walking long distances. Most people are genetically capable of doing this, even if they haven't done it much in their lifetime. I once read a book by a German called Theordore Illion, who disguised himself as a Tibetan and walked across Tibet at a time when Tibet was closed to foreigners, and he claimed to walk some staggering distances per day. "In Secret Tibet" was published in 1937, and is an interesting read. His follow up book had some stuff in it that was obviously made up, so I can't necessarily believe that the distances he claimed to have walked are true, but there is no doubt that he did a walk long way through Tibet and he did walk long distances each day.

I would say that the 8.0 mile walk I did on the Saturday was responsible for pulling my blood sugar numbers into the normal range on that day. On Saturday morning I also lifted some weights in my home gym. I did 160 forward wrist curls, 80 reverse wrist curls, 60 concentration curls, 20 single arm extensions, and 20 side bends. Those would have been done in the morning. I climbed 10 flights of stairs sometime on Saturday as well, and remember I was doing all this exercise to push down hard on my blood sugar levels. It seems to me looking back at this point that I must have spent a good part of that Saturday exercising.

Week Ending Sunday December 16, 2007

This week I walked 20.2 miles. Monday to Friday I walked 1.9 miles each night which is the standard walk we do to take the dog at night. On Sunday I walked 10.7 miles. I must have been working really hard to put pressure on my blood sugar levels because that is quite a distance. I can still walk 10 miles in a day if I wanted to, but it is not something I do now. That same week I climbed 130 flights of stairs at a little strip mall near where we live. That is equivalent to a climb of 1,820 feet. That week I did 760 forward wrist curls, 400 reverse wrist curls, 420 concentration curls, and 260 single arm extensions. I did double the number of single arm extensions I had done the previous week, but otherwise the weights lifted were about the same. I lifted weights for about

15 minutes each morning on Tuesday to Saturday. My blood sugar numbers for the week were as follows:

Monday 12-10-07, 6:30am 189 mg/dl (10.5 mmol/L)
Wednesday 12-12-07, 6:30pm 102 mg/dl (5.67 mmol/L) – after climbing 25 flights of stairs
Thursday 12-13-07, 6:12pm 106 mg/dl (5.89 mmol/L) – after climbing 25 flights of stairs
Thursday 12-13-07, 8:45pm 86 mg/dl (4.78 mmol/L) – after climbing another 25 flights of stairs = 50 flights of stairs for the night
Friday 12-14-07, 7:00pm 142 mg/dl (7.89 mmol/L) – no exercise at night
Saturday 12-15-07, 7:50am 154 mg/dl (8.56 mmol/L)
Sunday 12-16-07, 4:04pm 113 mg/dl (6.28 mmol/L)

Average reading for week ended 12-16-07 127 mg/dl (7.06 mmol/L)

The blood sugar numbers for this week give some incredibly valuable information. As you will see my blood sugar numbers were jumping all over the place. That stopped when I had things under control. I think the reason they are all over the place is that I was still draining my blood sugar reservoirs at this point. My feeling is that when they stabilized, which you will see a few weeks after this then at that point excess sugar in my bloodstream was being diverted to blood sugar reservoirs, whereas at this point in this week the excess blood sugar was just sitting in my bloodstream until I exercised it out, and you can see that on some days I was successful on exercising the sugar out of my bloodstream (with a lot of hard work), and other days I was not successful. Like I said in the main part of the book though, this is a war of attrition and at this point I was wearing my enemy down. I had breached his defenses in several places, but I hadn't gotten my army through the walls yet, and at night while I slept he was able to reassert himself to some extent.

I wrote the last paragraph at 11pm last night, and I have given this some thought overnight. When you see numbers jumping all over the place like this, with anything, it means that you are putting pressure on a tipping point, and that a flip into a different stable state is in the near future. My belief is that a type 2 diabetes state, and a non-type 2 diabetes state are both stable situations for the body, and once enough pressure is put on tipping points the body will flip into one state or the other. The heavy exercise was draining my blood sugar reserves, and putting strong pressure on the tipping point that would tip me out of type 2 diabetes. On the converse side, had I spent four hours a night sitting watching television I would have put massive pressure on a tipping point too, but it would have been a tipping point that would have flipped my body into a diabetes state. That, in effect, was what I had done all summer when I was working long hours and I was too tired to exercise and eat properly. I now know that the best way to get my body to relax after a long day at the office is to do a long walk or go stair climbing, and after time spent doing either exercise the stress just melts away. Television does not melt stress away, and one thing I do want to say is that the continual changing of the picture about once a second that they do now on American television probably pings the stress receptors, at least on men. The reason I believe this is that for most of our history mankind had to worry about being attacked, and taken down by large predators. This means that our bodies are trained to be alert to the slightest movement in our environments because that movement could be a large cat or a pack of wolves sneaking up on us. In the wild, the environment stays relatively stable until the moment before a big cat pounces, so changing the picture on the television every second pings that stress response like crazy. You may be sitting in the chair watching television, but a part of your mind is wondering whether it has to look for an escape route, and a mere few thousand years of living in cities and towns is not going to change that.

Let's look back over the blood sugar numbers for the week above now. I started the week with 189 mg/dl (10.5 mmol/L) on the morning of Monday 12-10-07. After having some numbers in range on Saturday that must have been a bit of a blow, and I can see that by the fact that I didn't take my blood sugar again until Wednesday evening. 189 mg/dl is quite a bit over the top of the limit, and I think that is closer to where my blood sugar naturally should have been at that point, and the lower numbers were caused by exercising hard and putting pressure on my blood sugar reservoirs. Don't forget that when you start this you have to use up not only the sugar in your bloodstream, but you also start with sugar storage reservoirs that are probably full. When I refer to sugar storage reservoirs, as I have said elsewhere, energy is not stored as glucose, fructose or sucrose, but as compounds that can be easily converted back to sugar and that is what you have to drain. Your body has sugar storage reserves all over the place, but if you attack like the Czarist Russian army from five sides at once then you will win, and your sugar storage reservoirs will lose.

I took my blood sugar again on Wednesday night at 6:30pm after climbing 25 flights of stairs and it was 102 mg/dl (5.67 mmol/L). Judging by the time I took my blood sugar I probably stopped on the way home from work, and climbed 25 flights of stairs before heading on home for dinner. I took my blood sugar again on Thursday night, but not in the morning, and this again is evidence that I really didn't want to see another high morning blood sugar reading. Here are the readings again and I took two readings which gives us some good information:

Thursday 12-13-07, 6:12pm 106 mg/dl (5.89 mmol/L) – after climbing 25 flights of stairs
Thursday 12-13-07, 8:45pm 86 mg/dl (4.78 mmol/L) – after climbing another 25 flights of stairs = 50 flights of stairs for the night

The amount of exercise I did Thursday night shows that I was really determined to beat this thing because I climbed 50 flights of stairs in two blocks of 25 flights. Now I had done a lot of stair climbing when we lived in Annapolis, Maryland, and I worked inside the Washington D.C. beltway, and I had done this to beat stress at the time. This was back around 2002, and at that point I would have been 43 years old. In 2007 when I did these exercises, I would have been 48 years old. I have to say again, do not try stair climbing without having your heart checked by your doctor first because it is an extremely strenuous exercise. My Scottish ancestry makes me a very determined man, and the more obstacles are put in my way, the harder I tend to push back. Sometimes I have surprised people who have been trying to manipulate me at work with this, and it is my belief that this world would be a lot more courteous if we had never ended dueling, and one man could still call another man out for swords or pistols at dawn.

The fact that I ramped up the exercise so hard this week was almost certainly due to having a morning blood sugar of 189 mg/dl (10.5 mmol/L) on the Monday, especially after having blood sugars in range on the Saturday two days before that. Now you will see this in your own numbers when you start attacking type 2 diabetes. Remember I said that this will be a war of attrition and that it will last eight weeks. Looking at the numbers in my spreadsheet, I actually beat type diabetes down in less than eight weeks, and remember every little bit of exercise you do will have an effect either on the sugar in your bloodstream or on your body's sugar storage reservoirs. Many of you may be unable to stair climb, but most of you will be able to walk, and you can build up to walking considerable distances. At the moment I walk 100 miles a month by taking five walks a week that add up to 25 miles a week. That takes me maybe an hour and a half a day. We all have crazy schedules these days, but you can work it in and like I have said before, exercise will de-stress you much better than many other activities. A good heavy exercise is running on the spot. In England I used to run on the spot for forty minutes just about every night, and I would put a CD on and listen to music while I did it. If Jacksonville has another extremely hot summer like last year then I will probably have to just give up on stair climbing in the summer, and switch to running on the spot or doing a lot of Tai Chi.

We can learn a lot from the two blood sugar readings taken on the Thursday night. The second reading was 86 mg/dl (4.78 mmol/L) and a doctor looking at that reading in isolation might say that I was looking in pretty good shape. Doctors are not stupid though and he or she would no doubt want to see a week of readings. This number of 86 mg/dl was the first reading I had gotten since the start of all this that was anywhere near the low end of the normal blood sugar range. Now the average of all the readings for that week was 127 mg/dl (7.06 mmol/L) but by sheer determination I had pulled one really good reading out of the hat, and despite the fact that my body had plenty of stored sugar available, I had overwhelmed it. The next night I did no exercise as it was a Friday night and I pulled in a blood sugar reading of 142 mg/dl (7.89 mmol/L) at 7:00pm. The following morning on

Saturday 12-15-07 at 7:50am the reading was 154 mg/dl (8.56 mmol/L).

This looks as though I put a lot of work in for nothing as it wasn't much lower than the reading on the Monday, but that is absolutely untrue because a few weeks later all my morning blood sugars were in the normal range. It is very likely that just having one reading of 86 mg/dl showed me that I could win. I took very little exercise on that Saturday. I did no walking or stair climbing. I did 70 forward wrist curls, 50 reverse wrist curls, 70 concentration curls and 60 single arm extensions. Sunday December 16 was a whole different ball game and I walked 10.7 miles and climbed 25 flights of stairs. The reading for Sunday 12-16-07 at 4:04pm was 113 mg/dl (6.28 mmol/L). Again here I pulled the number back into range by doing a lot of exercising, and all you can do at this point is to work hard, and aim to push one number here and one number there down into the limits. As you will see when we move ahead though, I started to get more and more numbers inside the range, and fairly quickly I arrived at the state where they were pretty much all in range. By the time we got to that point my army was in through the walls, and I had chased my enemy through his stronghold until my men were ready to gut him. That point is coming in a few weeks though, but my point is that a lot of the work was done here in this week with some real heavy exercise sessions.

Week Ending Sunday December 23, 2007

This was an interesting week because we flew to Aruba on Saturday December 22. I only had ten days vacation a year, which is pretty standard in America, and we all had to take a week off between Christmas and New Year's Day so I would usually take the family somewhere. This gives useful information though because although I could, and did, exercise while we were in Aruba I had very little control over what I ate. The food in Aruba was all cooked fresh though, and probably didn't have too many chemicals in it. The water in Aruba comes from a desalination plant and it is filtered over coral, and it tastes really good. While the British and French just do their best with rainfall on the islands they own in the Caribbean, the Dutch have made sure they never run out of water, at least on the Dutch islands I have been to.

We drove down to Fort Lauderdale on Friday December 21 as soon as I arrived home from work, which was a six hour drive from Jacksonville so this meant no exercise that night and none the night before as I had to pack. My exercise rates that week were really low, and again a change like this gives valuable information as it puts pressure back on the tipping points in the wrong direction, so let's get into the numbers and see what happened. I didn't do any walking that week until after we arrived in Aruba, and I walked 2 miles on Saturday 12-22-07, and 6 miles on Sunday 12-23-07. These are both estimates on the distances because I had no way to measure them, but on the Sunday my son and I went looking for a supermarket and it was a lot further away then we had been told. That week I only climbed 34 flights of stairs before we went to Aruba so I didn't do much there. I did 470 forward wrist curls, 330 reverse wrist curls, 190 concentration curls and 170 single arm extensions.

Let's have a look at my blood sugar records for that week now:

Monday 12-17-07, 6:42pm 117 mg/dl (6.50 mmol/L)
Tuesday 12-18-07, 6:25am 142 mg/dl (7.89 mmol/L)
Tuesday 12-18-07, 6:12pm 94 mg/dl (5.22 mmol/L)
Wednesday 12-19-07, 7:00 pm 108 mg/dl (6.0 mmol/L)
Thursday 12-20-07, 6:30am 112 mg/dl (6.22 mmol/L)
Thursday 12-20-07, 6:40 pm 94 mg/dl (5.22 mmol/L)
Sunday 12-23-07, 3:20pm 96 mg/dl (5.33 mmol/L)

Average reading for week ended 12-23-07 109 mg/dl (6.06 mmol/L)

The average reading for the week was 109 mg/dl (6.06 mmol/L), which was down from 127 mg/dl (7.06 mmol/L). I really didn't take much exercise this week but I must have drained my blood sugar reservoirs with all the exercise the previous week. The reason I can say that is because most of these blood sugar numbers are within the range. There are only two morning readings though and I suspect if I had taken more morning readings I would have more readings out of range. Having said that, on Thursday 12-20-

07 at 6:30am the reading was 112 mg/dl (6.22 mmol/L), which meant that I had the first morning blood sugar that was in range, and when I check my exercise records I did absolutely no exercise the night before. However, we can really see what happened by going to Aruba here because I wouldn't have another morning blood sugar in range until the morning of Monday 01-07-08 at 6:20am when it was 118 mg/dl (6.56 mmol/L). This is really valuable information because I think I had almost gotten things under control at this point, and had I exercised as hard during week ended December 23, 2007 as I did during the previous week ended December 16, 2007 then I might well have flipped my body out of a diabetes state that week. This is good though because it shows us the value of exercise and diet. I effectively took one to two weeks away from my normal schedule, as you will see by my exercise numbers, and my blood sugar numbers were driven higher by that. This shows that there is a time lag effect, and what I think happened here was that I drained my sugar storage reservoirs during the previous few weeks of heavy exercise. During week ended December 23, 2007 because the sugar storage had been drained somewhat, I suspect that some of the carbs I ate that week were diverted into my sugar storage reservoirs rather than pushing my blood sugar up. This is exactly how this works. Drain your sugar storage reservoirs and you have some leeway, and if you have some leeway then you have control. This is exactly like the example of the farmer from 4,000 years ago in the introduction. If I put pressure on the streams flowing onto his property, and I drain his reservoirs then pretty soon he starts to run out of water and his whole system is under pressure. That is exactly what we are doing here. I worked to drain my sugar storage reservoirs and because they were partially drained then I got away with not being able to exercise much during week ended December 23, 2007.

Let's break down the days of the week for week ended December 23, 2007 and do some analysis. The first number we have is Monday 12-17-07 at 6:42pm and that was 117 mg/dl (6.50 mmol/L). The only exercise I did on Monday was to climb 9 flights of stairs. I don't know why I only climbed 9 flights of stairs. That is in range but close to the top of the range and that probably impacted Tuesday morning's blood sugar number which was taken at 6:25am and was 142 mg/dl (7.89 mmol/L). On Tuesday I did

320 forward wrist curls, 230 reverse wrist curls, 190 concentration curls, and 120 single arm extensions. I also climbed 25 flights of stairs. I took my blood sugar again on Tuesday evening at 6:12pm and it was 94 mg/dl (5.22 mmol/L). This is a good number and on the evening of Wednesday 12-19-07 at 7:00 pm my blood sugar was 108 mg/dl (6.0 mmol/L). This is higher than the evening before but I did absolutely no exercise on Wednesday at all so I was able to pull in a reading that was in range. Given all the previous numbers, in my opinion, the only way I could have done that would be by draining my blood sugar reservoirs. I have two readings for the Thursday, a morning and evening and they are both in range:

Thursday 12-20-07, 6:30am 112 mg/dl (6.22 mmol/L)
Thursday 12-20-07, 6:40 pm 94 mg/dl (5.22 mmol/L)

Now this is really interesting because the reading on Thursday morning is only 4 mg/dl higher than the reading taken the night before. This is completely different from just a week or two before. If you look back over the numbers from earlier weeks my morning blood sugars were normally a good bit higher than my evening ones. That means there is progress there and this is why going to Aruba gives useful numbers because you can see the step back taken by not exercising. Friday and Saturday were involved in travelling and the next time I took my blood sugar was on Sunday 12-23-07 at 3:20pm and it was 96 mg/dl (5.33 mmol/L). This is a good number and I believe it was this low because my son and I had just walked 6 miles. This is a good end to the week in terms of blood sugar numbers. Contrast this number of 96 mg/dl (5.33 mmol/L) with the 293 mg/dl (16.28 mmol/L) at the test ordered by my doctor just two months earlier in late October 2007. One thing we should take into consideration too is that by this point I had lifted a lot of weights and this would mean that the glucose transporters in my muscles would have been stimulated a lot and that would mean they would be better at pulling sugar out of my blood than they had been before. Also muscle burns far more calories an hour than if there is no muscle there, or very little muscle there.

<u>Week Ending Sunday December 30, 2007 – Aruba</u>

Most of this week was spent in Aruba. We flew back on Saturday December 29, spent some time with friends in Fort Lauderdale and headed back home after that. Aruba was so hot it was hard to exercise and although I found some stairs and tried stair climbing it was just too hot to do it. I have been to the Portuguese island of Madeira off the coast of Morocco in Africa at latitude 32 degrees North, which is actually further north than I live now and I have been to the Hawaiian Islands several times and they are at a latitude of 19.6 North but Aruba in the depths of winter was hotter than either of them in the summer or so it felt.

All I managed to do in Aruba was walk. In the previous week I told you that my son and I walked 6 miles on the Sunday. Each day we were in Aruba I walked on the beach and I did 1.5 miles a day. This gave me 7.5 miles over 5 days and I walked 2.0 miles on Sunday December 30, so this gave me 9.5 miles for the week.

Wednesday 12-26-07, 7:20am 130 mg/dl (7.22 mmol/L)
Friday 12-28-07, 12:08pm 117 mg/dl (6.50 mmol/L)
Saturday 12-29-07, 6:44am 144 mg/dl (8.0 mmol/L)
Saturday 12-29-07, 10:01am 128 mg/dl (7.11 mmol/L)

Average reading for week ended 12-30-07 130 mg/dl (7.22 mmol/L)

You can see by the blood sugar numbers I have here that I started to slide back into type 2 diabetes during this week. Three out of four readings were out of range. What is missing from this is a really long walk. I have always felt that short walks don't drain your blood sugar reserves, but something like 5 miles does.

<u>Week Ending Sunday January 6, 2008</u>

There is always a danger for me in going on vacation because once I get out of my exercise routine it is hard to get back into it, and I can see it in the exercise records for this week. Just after this I went in really hard and the exercise records for week ended January 13 and January 20 show an enormous amount of work

174

done and I actually flipped myself out of type 2 diabetes sometime during week ended January 13. However, this is week ended January 6 so let's have a look at the numbers. I didn't do any walking at all until Saturday January 5, 2008 and on that day I walked 7.3 miles. On the Sunday I walked 5.1 miles making a total for the week of 12.4 miles. I didn't do any stair climbing until Sunday January 6 and I climbed 22 flights of stairs. I hardly lifted any weights that week either, I did 220 forward wrist curls, 80 reverse wrist curls, and 30 single arm extensions.

Let's have a look at the blood sugar readings now:

Monday 12-31-07, 6:27pm 113 mg/dl (6.28 mmol/L)
Wednesday 01-02-08, 6:07pm 97 mg/dl (5.39 mmol/L)
Thursday 01-03-08, 5:58am 128 mg/dl (7.11 mmol/L)
Thursday 01-03-08, 6:37pm 99 mg/dl (5.50 mmol/L)
Friday 01-04-08, 6:25am 142 mg/dl (7.89 mmol/L)
Friday 01-04-08, 7:06pm 113 mg/dl (6.28 mmol/L)
Saturday 01-05-08, (no time recorded) 92 mg/dl (5.11 mmol/L)
Sunday 01-06-08, 9:45am 131 mg/dl (7.28 mmol/L)
Sunday 01-06-08, 2:14pm 86 mg/dl (4.78 mmol/L)

Average reading for week ended 01-06-08 111 mg/dl (6.12 mmol/L)
Average reading for morning blood sugars 134 mg/dl (7.44 mmol/L)

I started to include the average morning blood sugar for the week here too because I copied those numbers out onto a separate tab on the spreadsheet and at the end of the day, good morning readings are what we are aiming at. The first thing I see when analyzing the data here is that all three morning readings were out of range. All the evening readings are inside the range. The two lowest were taken on Saturday and Sunday and it looks like I pushed these down by walking. On Saturday January 5, 2008 I walked 7.3 miles, and on Sunday I walked 5.1 miles making a total of 12.4 miles for the weekend. This gave me a blood sugar reading on Saturday of 92 mg/dl (5.11 mmol/L) and on Sunday of 86 mg/dl (4.78 mmol/L). On Sunday I did climb 22 flights of stairs as well. At this point, although I didn't yet realize it, I was about done with type 2 diabetes. After this date I only had two blood sugar readings that were over the limit in the next three months and both of them were literally just over with one at 127 mg/dl (7.06 mmol/L) on the morning of Tuesday January 29 and the other one on the morning of Tuesday February 12 at 130 mg/dl (7.22 mmol/L).

<u>Week Ending Sunday January 13, 2008</u>

This week I went in really hard with exercise and that is what you do. When victory is in sight you redouble your efforts and overwhelm your enemy and that is exactly what I did. My enemy, type 2 diabetes, started the week in a precarious position, and this is the week my army broke through his defenses, chased him down, and one of my soldiers smashed his head in with a mace and busted his jaw (a mace is a metal spiked ball on the end of a wooden shaft). However, type 2 diabetes is a tricky enemy, and whilst victory was mine this week, he can reincarnate and appear when you drop your guard so be aware of that. You must always do some exercise and you must always eat as little processed food as possible or you will find yourself staring him down again at a future date.

I focused very heavily on stair climbing this week and did very little walking and not much weight lifting although I was getting close to hitting weight lifting hard in the following week. This week I climbed 50 flights of stairs each night Monday to Thursday and 25 flights of stairs on Saturday and Sunday making a total for the week of 250 flights of stairs climbed. That equates to a height climbed of 3,500 feet. My main focus that week was on stair climbing. I walked 3.2 miles on Saturday and 1.9 miles on Sunday evening, although there is a note there that saying that rain prevented me from walking so there must have been a bad storm that day. That week I did 480 forward wrist curls, 370 reverse wrist curls, 50 concentration curls, 110 single arm extensions, and 60 bench presses.

That week I took my blood sugar a lot. I definitely did not realize at that point that I had already beaten type 2 diabetes and I was gearing up for a full scale assault on it together with full scale information gathering, which meant recording as many blood sugar readings as possible. That week I took 17 blood sugar readings which worked out to slightly more than two a day.

Monday 01-07-08, 6:20am 118 mg/dl (6.56 mmol/L)
Monday 01-07-08, 6:56pm 86 mg/dl (4.78 mmol/L)
Monday 01-07-08, 9:40pm 89 mg/dl (4.94 mmol/L)
Tuesday 01-08-08, 6:20am 109 mg/dl (6.06 mmol/L)
Tuesday 01-08-08, 6:48pm 93 mg/dl (5.17 mmol/L)
Tuesday 01-08-08, 9:25pm 103 mg/dl (5.72 mmol/L)
Wednesday 01-09-08, 6:22am 97 mg/dl (5.39 mmol/L)
Wednesday 01-09-08, 6:57pm 84 mg/dl (5.22 mmol/L)
Thursday 01-10-08, 6:25am 93 mg/dl (5.17 mmol/L)
Thursday 01-10-08, 7:30pm 89 mg/dl (4.94 mmol/L)
Friday 01-11-08, 6:18pm 90 mg/dl (5.0 mmol/L)
Saturday 01-12-08, 8:45am 114 mg/dl (6.33 mmol/L)
Saturday 01-12-08, 1:48pm 93 mg/dl (5.17 mmol/L)
Saturday 01-12-08, 5:54pm 90 mg/dl (5.0 mmol/L)
Sunday 01-12-08, 12:10am 100 mg/dl (5.56 mmol/L)
Sunday 01-12-08, 8:20am 108 mg/dl (6.0 mmol/L)
Sunday 01-12-08, 7:47pm 82 mg/dl (4.56 mmol/L)

Average reading for week ended 01-13-08 96 mg/dl (5.33 mmol/L)
Average reading for morning blood sugars 107 mg/dl (5.94 mmol/L)

The highest morning reading was on Monday 01-07-08 and was 118 mg/dl (6.56 mmol/L). Although this in range it is still quite high. However, this was the first week where all my morning blood sugars were in range, so it was a major step forward. I did no exercise on Friday night which may have resulted in Saturday morning being the second highest reading for the week. After this week I began to focus more on taking my blood sugar in the mornings because the real demonstration that you have things under control is when your morning blood sugar readings are all in range. I also kept a table showing what percentage of blood sugar readings were in the normal range. Week ending January 13, 2008 was the first week I had 100% of readings in range and after that apart from the two minor jumps that were just over 126 mg/dl in the morning everything was in range.

<u>Week Ending Sunday January 20, 2008</u>

This week I focused quite a bit on weight lifting. I started going to a gym at lunchtimes. This week I did 1,210 forward wrist curls, 660 reverse wrist curls, 150 concentration curls, 450 single arm extensions, 50 bench presses, and 240 dumbbell curls which work the biceps. At this point I was moving from using concentration curls, which are seated curls where the elbow is braced against the knee, to dumbbell curls which are done in a standing position. Weight lifting is important for the simple reason that it activates the GLUT 4 glucose transporters in your muscles, and the more responsive you can make these, the more they interact with insulin to pull sugar out of your bloodstream (see the chapter on Glucose Transporters).

I only did about half as many flights of stairs as the week before. I climbed 105 flights of stairs for the week which was a total height gain of 1,470 feet. This week I walked 4.3 miles on Friday and 3.2 miles on Sunday. There is a big gap in exercise in the evenings for Tuesday, Wednesday and Thursday. I may well have worked late those evenings because it was at this point we realized that the recession in the United States was really beginning to bite, and we needed to change our business strategy to cope with this. Here are the blood sugar numbers for the week:

Monday 01-14-08, 6:22am 114 mg/dl (6.33mmol/L)
Tuesday 01-15-08, 6:27am 96 mg/dl (5.33 mmol/L)
Wednesday 01-16-08, 6:24am 93 mg/dl (5.17 mmol/L)
Thursday 01-17-08, 6:23am 93 mg/dl (5.17 mmol/L)
Friday 01-18-08, 1:04pm 80 mg/dl (4.44 mmol/L)
Friday 01-18-08, 5:45pm 79 mg/dl (4.39 mmol/L)
Saturday 01-19-08, 8:50am 110 mg/dl (6.11 mmol/L)

Average reading for week ended 01-20-08 94 mg/dl (5.22 mmol/L)
Average reading for morning blood sugars 101 mg/dl (5.61 mmol/L)

These are mostly morning readings and the first thing that springs out is that the Monday morning reading is high again which illustrates definitely that easing back on exercise and eating at restaurants over the weekend tended to push my blood sugar up. I didn't eat anything like a dessert or anything with sugar in although there may easily have been hidden sugar in the restaurant food. I always avoid things like teriyaki sauces, and other sauces that are sweetened. I didn't do any stair climbing or walking on Wednesday night or Thursday night. Thursday morning's reading was 93 mg/dl (5.17 mmol/L), so even though I didn't exercise the night before I had a good morning reading. I will do one more week as my blood sugars were now in range, and after I have done that week I will do a listing of the average morning readings for the weeks after that.

Week Ending Sunday January 27, 2008

The first thing to note here is that our wedding anniversary is January 22 and I have a note on the exercise spreadsheet that we went down to Disney in Orlando over the weekend. We probably drove down on the Friday night and that would explain why the last blood sugar reading was done on Thursday night. This week I climbed 78 flights of stairs and this was down because we were going away. The week after that I pushed the stairs back up to 150 flights of stairs. This week I only walked 1.9 miles on Monday night although I would have walked a lot at Disney as it is usually 6 miles round each park, and I also walk around the lake where we stay. That weekend we stayed at the Coronado Springs resort, and Cecilia's brother Marty came over to see us on the Sunday before we left. I did lift quite a lot of weights that week. I did 1,350 forward wrist curls, 650 reverse wrist curls, 20 concentration curls, 760 single arm extensions, 50 bench presses, and 230 dumbbell curls. Here are my blood sugar numbers for the week:

Monday 01-21-08, 6:25am 107 mg/dl (5.94 mmol/L)
Monday 01-21-08, 6:47pm 92 mg/dl (5.11 mmol/L)
Monday 01-21-08, 10:02pm 91 mg/dl (5.06 mmol/L)
Tuesday 01-22-08, 6:15am 102 mg/dl (5.67 mmol/L)

Wednesday 01-23-08, 6:10am 101 mg/dl (5.61 mmol/L)
Thursday 01-24-08, 6:20am 98 mg/dl (5.44 mmol/L)
Thursday 01-24-08, 7:04pm 91 mg/dl (5.06 mmol/L)

Average reading for week ended 01-27-08 97 mg/dl (5.39 mmol/L)
Average reading for morning blood sugars 102 mg/dl (5.67 mmol/L)

The Monday morning reading this week was 107 mg/dl (5.94 mmol/L), which was better. I'm not going to go on listing blood sugars week by week here, although I will give you the averages. My Monday morning readings were often the highest of the week, which I believe was caused by eating at restaurants over the weekend. I did have some Monday readings in the low 100s, and I had one in the 90s. My average morning reading for the weeks tended to be in the low 100s as you will see below. This is technically classed as pre-diabetic, but I'll take those numbers over a morning number of 293 mg/dl (16.28 mmol/L) any day, which was where I was when I started this fight. In one of the weeks below you will see the morning average jump up to 112 mg/dl (6.22 mmol/L). I looked at this, and it was caused by a series of high morning numbers, but tucked away in there on Friday February 15, 2008 was a morning reading of 85 mg/dl (4.72 mmol/L), which was actually a great morning reading. That is weird because it is the day after Valentine's Day, and I didn't take any exercise the night before, and we also must have gone out to eat.

Well here you have it. This is a step by step progression out of diabetes. As I have said before, I am just an ordinary man. There is nothing I have done that you cannot do. Attack from five sides like the Russian army of the Czars, and you will destroy your enemy, as they destroyed theirs. Your weapons are walking, a heavy exercise, and weight lifting, which makes three sides of the attack. A fourth weapon is control of what you eat, with an emphasis on complex carbohydrates and raw food whenever you can do it. The fifth side of the attack is an attitude of quiet determination. A quietly determined man, or woman, is often unstoppable when they put their mind to something. I will copy the morning average readings for weeks ended February 3, 2008 to March 23, 2008 for you to look at below.

Week ending 02-03-08; average morning reading 103 mg/dl (5.72 mmol/L)
Week ending 02-10-08; average morning reading 103 mg/dl (5.72 mmol/L)
Week ending 02-17-08; average morning reading 112 mg/dl (6.22 mmol/L)
Week ending 02-24-08; average morning reading 106 mg/dl (5.89 mmol/L)
Week ending 03-02-08; average morning reading 104 mg/dl (5.78 mmol/L)
Week ending 03-09-08; average morning reading 104 mg/dl (5.78 mmol/L)
Week ending 03-16-08; average morning reading 105 mg/dl (5.83 mmol/L)
Week ending 03-23-08; average morning reading 94 mg/dl (5.22 mmol/L)

There are no results for week ending March 30, 2008, and there is a note about going on a trip to Georgia with work, and coming back tired from the trip. The next few weeks I appear to have been taking readings sporadically, and it looks like things were probably getting a little crazy at work with the recession looming. If you look at the weeks I do have above though what you can see is a man who has won his battle with type 2 diabetes. You will always see that in the morning numbers. You can do what I have done and I will close Appendix 1 with this message:

Now is the time for you to face type 2 diabetes on the battlefield. Remember that you will win, and he will lose. Unlock your weapons, ride forward into battle, and remember that you ride with Vikings. Good luck and Godspeed.

Blood Sugar Converter

The following link will give you a converter that will convert US blood sugar numbers to UK blood sugar numbers:

http://www.diabetes.co.uk/blood-sugar-converter.html

The range classed as the normal blood sugar range in the United States is 80 mg/dl to 126 mg/dl.

Here are some of the main numbers:

80 mg/dl is equivalent to 4.44 mmol/L
126 mg/dl is equivalent to 7.0 mmol/L
150 mg/dl is equivalent to 8.33 mmol/L
200 mg/dl is equivalent to 11.11 mmol/L
250 mg/dl is equivalent to 13.89 mmol/L
300 mg/dl is equivalent to 16.67 mmol/L

The Dynamind Technique

The Dynamind Technique was developed by Serge Kahili King, from Hawaii. To quote Serge's own words:

"The Dynamind Technique is based on a theory that all physical, emotional and mental problems are related to excessive tension in the body. The theory proposes that tension accumulates in layers, with focal points that produce specific symptoms. Healing takes place when tension layers are relaxed."

In my opinion, this is well worth trying. It takes just a few minutes, and costs you nothing, so give it a try. I said elsewhere in this book, that when I began to investigate the things in the world that science chose to ignore, I found a mixture of things that worked, and things that did not. Everything I have tried from Serge King's books has worked, and some of those things that have worked, cannot be explained by Western science. I don't know Serge King, and I have never met him, but I am a great believer that if something works, then that knowledge should be passed on.

Here is the link to Serge King's Dynamind Technique:

http://www.alohainternational.org/html/dmteng.html

A Note on the Author

Michael Ward was born in Glasgow, Scotland, grew up in Nottingham, England and moved to Alaska when he was 37 years old. He was a single father for six years in England and his son moved to America with him. Michael has worked inside the Washington Beltway as an engineer and now lives with his family in Florida. As well as being the author of "Type 2 Diabetes: How to Kick its Ass", he is the author of one Scandinavian crime novel, four books of short stories, the Lisa Molin Assassin series, the Stephen Haggerty Assassin series, the Dangerous Scotsman series and The Beach at the End of Time series.

In total Michael has 44 books/short stories out on Amazon and Barnes and Noble. Many of them are ebooks but Michael will be putting more out as print-on-demand books through Create Space on Amazon.